D0780956

Overcoming
Hearing Aid
Fears

Overcoming
Hearing Aid
Fears *The Road to*
Better Hearing

JOHN M. BURKEY

Rutgers University Press

New Brunswick, New Jersey, and London

Library of Congress Cataloging-in-Publication Data

Burkey, John M., 1959–
Overcoming hearing aid fears : the road to better hearing / John M. Burkey.
p. cm.
Includes bibliographical references and index.
ISBN 0-8135-3309-0 (hardcover : alk. paper) — ISBN 0-8135-3310-4 (pbk. : alk. paper)
1. Hearing aids—Popular works.   I. Title.
RF300 .B87 2003
617.8'9-dc21

2003000432

British Cataloging-in-Publication information is available from the British Library.

Manufactured in the United States of America

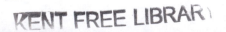

Contents

Illustrations

Acknowledgments

I wish to thank Audra Wolfe, Ph.D., science editor, and Adi Hovav, editorial assistant, at Rutgers University Press for their insightful comments and suggestions during the preparation of this book. Expert copyediting was provided by Debbie Self. I also wish to thank the physicians, audiologists, nurses, and support staff of the Lippy Group for Ear, Nose, and Throat for their encouragement throughout this project. Finally, I wish to thank my wife, Karen, for her love and understanding during the writing and publication of this book.

I've had the privilege to work with and help many people with hearing loss. Some of their stories are included in this book. All of the names of patients given are pseudonyms; thereby no breach of patient confidentiality has been committed.

Overcoming
Hearing Aid
Fears

Introduction

Cindy Johnson was forty-eight years old when I first saw her as a patient. She had worked for many years as an outside sales representative for a large corporation. Although she could easily understand loud speech, she struggled when speech was at a normal conversational level. She could not understand speech that was soft. Although Cindy recognized that the hearing loss was affecting her work and her personal life, she had avoided an evaluation because she feared this would lead to her having to wear hearing aids. Her main concern was that hearing aids would make her appear old. She had suffered her hearing loss for several years until a new boyfriend whom she cared about very much convinced her that the hearing loss was affecting their relationship and that she should seek help.

Cindy's hearing evaluation confirmed the hearing loss and indicated that she would be a good candidate for hearing aids. She purchased a hearing aid for each ear and adjusted to them quickly. She was thrilled that she could again hear and understand her clients at work. The hearing aids made it easier to talk with her boyfriend and allowed her to feel more comfortable and confident talking with him and others in most settings. By allowing her to do more comfortably, the hearing aids helped her to feel younger rather than older. She wears her hearing aids every day and would now not be without them.

Florence Hamilton was an eighty-one-year-old widow who was brought to my office by her daughter for a hearing evaluation. She had suffered a stroke several years previously that had left her with paralysis on the left side. She moved in with her daughter following her stroke. Although Mrs. Hamilton denied any significant hearing problem, her daughter reported that the television was uncomfortably loud and everyone had to speak loudly or directly into her mother's ear to be understood. Complicating matters was the fact that Mrs. Hamilton had macular degeneration. She could not use her vision to make up for what she could not hear. Hearing tests confirmed that Mrs. Hamilton had a significant hearing loss in both ears. Although she was not convinced that her hearing was bad enough for a hearing aid, Mrs. Hamilton agreed to try an aid for the right ear. After one month of use, Mrs. Hamilton had become very comfortable wearing her hearing aid but stated that she was still unsure whether or not it was necessary. Her daughter countered that the hearing aid was indeed necessary and that the family had enjoyed a whole month with the television at a comfortable volume and that no one had to yell to be heard. After three months of use, Mrs. Hamilton readily acknowledged that the aid was a great help. She could now hear and understand the people who always seemed to be mumbling before she wore the aid. She was putting it on the first thing every morning and asked her daughter to find it for her if she could not see where it had been placed the night before.

These examples show that people can ultimately benefit from hearing aids even if they are slow to accept their hearing loss or resistant to the idea of wearing hearing aids. Mrs. Hamilton did not realize how much she was affected by her hearing loss until she tried a hearing aid and experienced the improvement. Miss Johnson acknowledged her hearing loss but would not have overcome her resistance to wearing hearing aids without outside encouragement. Having someone to provide help and encouragement was one of the most important factors for each of these people to become successful hearing aid users. In contrast, many people with hearing loss do not even try hearing aids. They refuse to acknowledge their hearing problem or are crippled by their hearing aid fears.

The exact number of people who suffer hearing loss is unknown. The most cited statistic regarding the prevalence of hearing loss in the United States is from the National Institute on Deafness and Other Communication Disorders (1989). The institute estimated that twenty-eight million people, or approximately 10 percent of the United States population, are hearing impaired. Other reports have generally agreed with this percentage (Kochkin 1990; Kochkin 1993; Kochkin 1996; Ries 1994). Assuming a global population of approximately six billion, this could equate to six hundred million people with hearing loss worldwide.

As a group, the elderly are the most likely to suffer hearing loss. A recent study from the Centers for Disease Control reports that one-third of people seventy years of age or older are hearing impaired (Desai et al. 2001). They reported that while people sixty-five years of age and older comprise only 12.8 percent of the population, they account for 37 percent of those with hearing losses. The percentage of people with hearing loss increases from one-fourth for people aged seventy to seventy-four years to one-half for people eighty-five years of age or older. The total number of hearing-impaired persons is expected to increase dramatically in the next few years due to aging of the baby-boom generation and increasing longevity.

Other characteristics associated with a higher-than-average incidence of hearing loss are being of Caucasian ancestry, having under twelve years of education, having family income under ten thousand dollars per year, and performing service or blue-collar work (Ries 1994). This report also noted a greater likelihood of hearing loss in men than in women. The size of this difference increased with age. The rate of hearing loss for men in the labor force has been reported to be twice that of working women (Collins and Thornberry 1989). This difference may have a greater association with a person's specific vocation, however, than with gender. Women who worked at blue-collar industrial jobs such as machine operator or assembler were on average 40 percent more likely to have a hearing loss than other working women (Collins and Thornberry 1989).

The hearing losses discussed in the above reports are severe enough to interfere with a person's ability to hear or communicate with others. These are not the slight hearing losses that might show up on a hearing test but go unnoticed by the person involved. These are hearing losses that affect people's lives. The majority of the hearing losses are sensorineural (nerve) losses that cannot be medically or surgically corrected. The best available option for these millions is to use hearing aids to compensate for the problem. Unfortunately, the most common feeling regarding this option is "Anything but hearing aids!"

A 1997 study of assistive technology devices from the National Center for Health Statistics reported that fewer than five million people in the United States use hearing aids (Russell et al. 1997). Other reviews report that only 23 percent of the people who could benefit from hearing aids actually own them (Kochkin 1993; Weinstein 1996).

There are numerous reasons why people do not want hearing aids, but the end result of this attitude is that few of the people who could be helped by this technology actually are. The rest suffer their hearing loss. The loss affects their careers, their personal lives, and their social interactions. Often, the hearing loss negatively affects their self-esteem, and social withdrawal or depression is the result.

Hearing loss is a quality-of-life issue. In a hearing world, good hearing is often required for a person to participate fully. Hearing loss can limit a person's options. It can prevent a person from satisfying his or her wants and needs. From early morning until late at night, a person uses hearing. It is one of only five senses available through which a person can experience the world. Hearing is used more than any other sense in communicating with others.

Hearing loss can prevent a person from being able to hear the birds sing in the morning or hear the wind blow through the trees. It can eliminate the joy a person might experience from conversing with friends or loved ones. It can limit a person's ability to use the telephone. It affects every aspect of a person's life where there is a need to hear.

Friends and family are also affected. It is not just a matter of watching the person suffer with a hearing loss. Any shared activities that become limited for the person with hearing loss also become limited for the friends and family of this person. The person with hearing loss is frustrated that he or she cannot do many of the things he or she used to do. Friends and family are frustrated that they no longer have a partner with whom they can do these things. Everyone suffers.

The National Council on Aging (2000) issued a report titled "The Consequences of Untreated Hearing Loss in Older Persons." The study found that people with an untreated hearing loss were more likely to experience sadness and depression, worry and anxiety, paranoia, reduced social activity, and emotional turmoil and insecurity than their peers. Older individuals who used hearing aids were more likely to report better relationships with their families, better feelings about themselves, improved mental health, and greater independence and security than did others of the same age group who did not use hearing aids.

A randomized study of the hearing impaired (Mulrow, Aguilar, Endicott, Tuley et al. 1990) found that 82 percent of the participants reported that hearing loss had an adverse effect on their quality of life. Reported adverse effects included depression, communication problems, social and emotional difficulties, and reduced cognitive function. A related study (Mulrow, Aguilar, Endicott, Velez et al. 1990) found that the majority of people reported these difficulties even when there was only a mild to moderate hearing loss. Confirmation of these negative effects is not confined, however, to the person with hearing loss. Brooks and associates (2001) found that significant others of a hearing-impaired partner experienced not only communication difficulties, but also increased difficulties in personal and social relationships.

Mulrow, Aguilar, Endicott, Tuley, and colleagues (1990) concluded that the negative effects associated with hearing loss were reversible with hearing aids. Another study suggested that hearing aids could be used to help protect against the development of cognitive impairment and disability in the elderly (Cacciatore et al. 1999). Mulrow et al. (1992) additionally found that the improvements in communication, mood, and social and emotional health were long term.

The purpose of this book is to help people to keep hearing loss from affecting their quality of life. Basic information on the function of a normal ear is provided first as a reference. Discussed next is the hearing-impaired ear and how a hearing aid helps to compensate for this damage.

One of the initial steps in overcoming a hearing loss is to examine the attitudes and beliefs that often stand in the way of a person obtaining or using hearing aids. Refusing to believe that there is a hearing problem is the first of these beliefs. This problem is discussed in the chapter "Denial and Acceptance of Hearing Loss." The chapters "Appearance and Deeper Concerns," "Fears and Doubts," and "Cost" address other obstacles that prevent people from benefiting from hearing aids.

Other chapters provide specific examples of the benefits of wearing hearing aids and of problems that are avoided when a person wears hearing aids. The impact of a person's hearing aid use on friends and family is also examined. Amid the numerous hearing-aid-related concerns and fears that people express, it is sometimes easy for them to forget that the goal is to be able to hear. Examples highlight some of the situations in which hearing-impaired persons or their families feel that trying to compensate for hearing loss is a worthwhile goal.

In the chapter titled "Hearing Aids 101," I provide basic information about the different hearing aid styles and circuitry options for anyone who is considering hearing aid use. This chapter also includes consumer-related issues like purchasing hearing aids on a trial basis and choosing between basic and more expensive models. Although a lifetime of hearing aid commercials and advertisements may provide the most common education for people considering hearing aids, it is not necessarily the optimal preparation.

In "Rejoining the Hearing World" I reveal a game plan for anyone who wants to try hearing aids. The steps include recognizing the hearing loss, confronting hearing-aid-related concerns, finding a hearing aid professional, selecting hearing aids, and then trying and successfully using hearing aids. Practical information at each step is provided for the person with hearing loss and also for family or friends who may want to help.

The discussions about hearing aids that are included in this book are based on my experience as a clinical audiologist evaluating and caring for more than fifty thousand patients with hearing loss. Each issue addressed was a concern of a real patient, a relative, or a friend. The majority of concerns expressed were repeated by patient after patient. In clinical practice it is possible to help a person work through these concerns so that he or she can compensate for his or her hearing loss and have an improved quality of life. This guide is intended to pass along knowledge derived from my clinical practice to you, the readers. This information can help a person with hearing loss address and work through his or her own hearing aid concerns. It can also help friends and family of a person with hearing loss. It is my hope that friends and family will use this information to understand the person's situation better and to help them take steps to overcome it.

1 Medical Observations on the Normal, Impaired, and Aided Ear

The Normal Ear

The human auditory system is extremely sensitive. Sound waves that displace the eardrum less than the width of a hair are clearly detectable. A normal ear can process frequencies ranging from twenty to twenty thousand cycles per second. It can process speech that is softer than a person could whisper or louder than a person could yell. The ear can also detect subtle variations in pitch, loudness, and intonation. It can do all of this effectively without conscious effort.

The human ear is divided into three parts: the outer ear, the middle ear, and the inner ear (see fig. 1.1).

The Outer Ear

The outer ear consists of the outer part we can see (the auricle), the external ear canal, and the eardrum (tympanic membrane). The purpose of the outer ear is to collect sound and focus it into the ear. The ear canal is generally about an inch in length and one-fourth inch in diameter. Cartilage covered by skin forms the outer half of the ear canal. The inner half of the canal is made up of skin covering the bone of the skull. In addition to carrying sound further into the ear, the ear canal shapes sound. The resonance of the canal favors the high pitches that are important to understand many consonants in the spoken word.

The Middle Ear

The middle ear is an air-filled cavity. It is bordered on the outside by the eardrum and on the inside by the inner ear. The middle ear space has a volume of one or two cubic centimeters. It is in this space that the middle ear bones rest. The outermost bone is the malleus. The

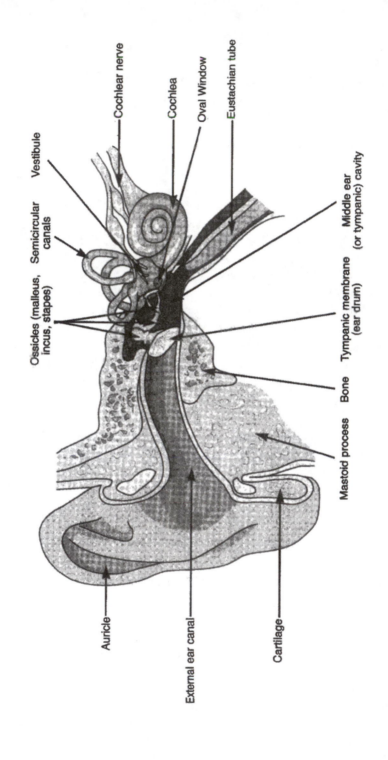

Cochlear nerve

Cochlea

Oval Window

Eustachian tube

Vestibule

Semicircular canals

Middle ear (or tympanic) cavity

Ossicles (malleus, incus, stapes)

Tympanic membrane (ear drum)

Bone

Mastoid process

Auricle

External ear canal

Cartilage

center bone is the incus, and the innermost bone is the stapes. These middle ear bones are also referred to as the hammer, the anvil, and the stirrup. Collectively, they are called the ossicles. The malleus attaches to the eardrum on one end of the ossicular chain. On the other end of the chain, the footplate of the stapes bone connects to the inner ear through a small opening between the middle and inner ear called the oval window.

The purpose of the middle ear is to prevent a loss in power as sound is transferred from the outside air to the fluids in the inner ear. The importance of this function cannot be understated. People who swim underwater can attest to how little sound reaches them when a person on the surface is speaking. The majority of sound is lost as the sound waves move from the air to the water. Just as much sound can be lost making the transition from air to the fluids in the inner ear. The middle ear overcomes this power loss in two ways. A small amount of the transition is overcome by the ossicles working in a lever action. More important is the size difference between the eardrum and the stapes bone. The eardrum has a much larger surface area than the footplate of the stapes. This allows sound to be collected across the entire surface of the eardrum and focused into the inner ear.

One other structure of note involving the middle ear is the Eustachian tube. This is a small passageway leading from the front of the middle ear into an area behind the nasal cavity and the back portion of the roof of the mouth. It is this tube that allows the ear to equalize pressure as you change elevation or dive underwater.

The Inner Ear

The inner ear is important for hearing and balance. The balance portion of the ear is called the vestibular system. It is made up of three semicircular canals and the vestibule. The structures of the vestibular system are fluid filled and work by detecting the movement of this fluid as a person changes position. The semicircular canals are responsible for detecting rotational movement. The vestibule contains the utricle and saccule that detect linear acceleration. A per-

Figure 1.1. (opposite)   The human ear. Courtesy of the Society of Otorhinolaryngology and Head-Neck Nurses (www.sohnnurse.com).

son's instinctive sense of up and down is provided by the vestibular system detecting the force that gravity exerts on the fluids within the system.

The portion of the inner ear responsible for hearing is called the cochlea. This is also a fluid-filled structure. The cochlea appears snail shaped and has approximately two and one-half turns. It contains the sensory nerves responsible for hearing. Each ear contains thousands of these nerves that are aligned along the length of the cochlea in a structure called the organ of Corti. The purpose of these sensory cells is to convert the mechanical motion of the fluid in the inner ear into an electrical signal that can be sent to the brain along the cochlear nerve. Each sensory cell has a small hair (cilia) that extends from the top and detects movement. As sound waves move the fluid in the inner ear, a shearing force is exerted across the cilia that activate the cell. The mechanical properties of the inner ear cause the nerve cells to be tuned to specific frequencies. The cells at the base of the cochlea where sound enters the ear are tuned for high-frequency sounds. Sensory cells further along the organ of Corti are tuned for progressively lower frequencies.

The Hearing-Impaired Ear

The ear is a complex system in which there is much that can go wrong. If something does go awry, hearing loss is the usual result. A hearing loss is confirmed or ruled out through a short battery of standardized tests called an audiologic evaluation. The testing usually takes fifteen to twenty minutes and is painless. The person being tested either presses a button or raises a hand whenever a beeping sound is heard through headphones. This provides a measure of the quietest sound a person can hear across a range of frequencies. The person being tested is also asked to repeat words. Some of the words will get very soft in order to determine the quietest level that the words can be recognized. Another list of words is presented at a louder level. The patient repeats these words also, but the goal here is to provide a measure of the clarity of hearing. The test results are comparable from one person to another and repeatable over time because the test equipment is calibrated to a national standard and the words are from standardized lists.

The causes of hearing loss are many. A few of the causes would include earwax, infection, disease, circulatory problems, trauma, noise exposure, toxic medications, and heredity or hereditary weakness. Although the exact cause of some hearing losses is never known, it is important to try to discern the cause to prevent the possibility of further damage. Knowing the cause, however, does not always serve as the most practical system for classifying hearing loss. A good example of this would be hearing losses caused by trauma. Depending on the type and severity of the trauma, the outer, middle, or inner ear could be damaged. Two or all three parts of the ear could be affected, and the amount of damage could be different in each part.

A more practical system is to classify hearing loss based on the part of the ear that is damaged. This provides a simpler classification that can always be determined. It also provides an indication of whether the hearing loss is permanent or medically treatable because management and prevention options vary according to the type and placement of the damage.

The three primary classifications of hearing loss are conductive, sensorineural, and mixed.

Conductive Hearing Loss

A hearing loss is termed *conductive* when it affects the structures that normally conduct sound to the inner ear. This includes both the outer and middle ear. The cause of a conductive hearing loss can be as simple as earwax blocking the ear canal. Sound can also be blocked by fluid or infection in the middle ear. Other common causes for a conductive hearing loss are a ruptured eardrum or damage to the middle ear bones.

An attribute shared by most conductive hearing losses is that they are usually medically treatable. An audiologist, a nurse, or a physician can remove wax that is blocking an ear canal. The wax might instead be eliminated through the use of an over-the-counter ear wash. A physician can treat infection in the ear with antibiotics or drain fluid from the middle ear with a procedure called a myringotomy. A torn eardrum may be patched or reconstructed, and damaged middle ear bones can often be replaced with a prosthesis. A person's hearing is usually restored completely or in part once any blockage is cleared or damage is repaired.

Sensorineural Hearing Loss

A hearing loss is termed *sensorineural* when it affects the sensory cells in the inner ear. The severity of a sensorineural hearing loss depends on the amount of nerve damage—the greater the damage, the greater the hearing loss. In addition to affecting the sensitivity or loudness of hearing, a sensorineural hearing loss can also affect the clarity of hearing. Even when loud enough, speech may not always be understandable.

Most people will develop at least some sensorineural hearing loss as they age. Noise exposure is another common cause of sensorineural hearing loss. Often, multiple factors are responsible. Sometimes the cause is never known. With very few exceptions, sensorineural hearing losses are permanent. The best that can be done is to compensate for the loss with hearing aids.

Mixed Hearing Loss

A mixed hearing loss occurs when a conductive and a sensorineural hearing loss are present in the same ear. A person can have wax in the ear canal blocking incoming sounds and also have sensorineural hearing loss from aging. Similarly, a person could have a sensorineural hearing loss from years of noise exposure and experience added hearing difficulties due to an infection in this same ear. The prognosis for a mixed loss is identical to that of its components. The conductive portion can usually be treated medically, but the sensorineural portion will remain.

The Aided Ear

The hope exists that it may one day be possible to regrow or regenerate damaged hearing nerves and thus eliminate most hearing losses and the need for hearing aids. Because some animals naturally regenerate hearing nerve cells, there is the hope that a medicine or treatment will be found to allow humans to do this also. It is not realistic, however, to plan on this as an alternative to hearing aids. Doing so is similar to buying lottery tickets as a retirement plan.

Hearing aids are an effective way to compensate for hearing losses that are not medically correctable. The basic concept of how a hearing aid works is fairly simple (see fig. 1.2). Sound waves enter the hearing aid and vibrate the diaphragm of the microphone. The microphone converts this mechanical energy into an electrical signal that is sent to the amplifier. The amplifier selectively increases the strength of this signal by frequency based on a person's individual hearing loss. The hearing aid user can then turn this strengthened and shaped signal louder or softer based on listening needs or comfort. The signal is sent to the receiver, which acts as a little speaker. It converts the electrical signal back into sound waves and directs this sound down the ear canal toward the eardrum.

It is common knowledge that hearing aids can be used to compensate for a hearing loss. There are a number of medical concerns and misunderstandings, however, that can cause people to incorrectly conclude that hearing aids would not be of help for them. These medical concerns fall into the categories of misunderstanding what hearing aids can and cannot do, concern that they may cause health problems, or that they might cause pain or discomfort.

What Hearing Aids Can and Cannot Do

I didn't think hearing aids would help a sensorineural hearing loss.
Hearing aids compensate well for mild or moderate sensorineural hearing losses. When the amount of nerve damage in the inner ear is limited, the clarity of hearing usually remains fairly good. Primarily, the volume needs to be increased enough to bring the softer sounds to a level that is audible.

Hearing aids can also be used to compensate for more severe hearing losses. The increased amount of nerve damage in the ear, however, is likely to cause some imprecise processing of sound. A severe sensorineural hearing loss can also make it difficult to get soft sounds loud enough to be heard without other sounds being uncomfortably loud. Hearing aids still help in this case, but they can-

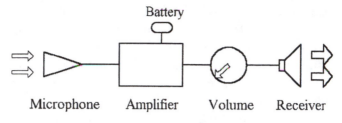

Figure 1.2. Block diagram of a simple hearing aid.

not completely compensate for the loss. This fact is surely the basis of the belief that hearing aids cannot correct for sensorineural hearing loss. If you tried to have a conversation with someone with this sort of damage with and without hearing aids, however, you could quickly tell the difference.

I thought hearing aids would only help a sensorineural hearing loss. While some people may incorrectly conclude that hearing aids cannot overcome the communication difficulties caused by a sensorineural hearing loss, others incorrectly conclude that this is the only type of hearing loss that hearing aids can help.

In the few instances where the mechanical damage in the middle ear is too severe to repair or when the person's overall health is too uncertain for surgery to be attempted, hearing aids remain an option. Unlike the distortion or loss of clarity that result from nerve damage, conductive hearing losses simply attenuate sound. The impairment acts as a wall that the sound has to pass through. Wearing a hearing aid forces sound through this wall to the hearing nerves in the inner ear. The person then hears well and clearly.

The kinds of hearing aids used with a conductive hearing loss are not usually physically different from those that would be used with a sensorineural hearing loss. The algorithm used to program the hearing aids, however, is slightly different. The one exception is a bone conduction hearing aid that is worn behind the ear rather than in the ear. This is used when the conductive hearing loss is caused by the congenital absence of an ear canal or when chronic infection would prevent the use of a traditional hearing aid.

Hearing aids can also be helpful when there is a mixed hearing loss. If the conductive portion of the hearing loss can be medically or surgically eliminated, then a smaller- and milder-gain hearing aid can be worn to compensate for the remaining sensorineural hearing loss. If the conductive portion cannot be corrected, then a more powerful hearing aid is used to overcome both parts of the hearing loss.

I thought hearing aids would not help hearing losses caused by noise exposure.

It is commonly believed that people who have lost their hearing through noise exposure cannot wear hearing aids. Like the belief that hearing aids cannot correct sensorineural hearing loss or can correct only sensorineural hearing loss, this view is incorrect.

A noise-induced hearing loss is just a special type of sensorineural hearing loss. As with all sensorineural hearing losses the damage is in the tiny nerve cells within the inner ear. The loud sounds so overpower the delicate mechanisms in the ear that some of the hearing nerves are destroyed. Most damage usually occurs in the hearing nerves for high frequencies, but with long-term noise exposure, the hearing at all frequencies can be affected. This pattern of damage occurs regardless of whether the damaging noise was from factory work, firearms, music, or other recreational activity. Earplugs or earmuffs can prevent this hearing loss from occurring, but once the nerves are damaged they are not medically repairable.

Hearing aids are actually the best way to compensate for hearing losses caused by noise exposure. In addition to increasing the overall volume of sounds, the hearing aids can emphasize the high frequencies where the loss is greatest. This lets a person hear the different pitches more evenly. This is particularly helpful for understanding women and children who have higher-pitched voices. Without hearing aids, women and children are typically the greatest listening challenge for a person with a noise-induced loss.

Do I really need two hearing aids?

It is not necessarily true that a person must have two hearing aids. Rather, a person will do better with two hearing aids. There are several reasons for this.

The first advantage to wearing two hearing aids is that it will be easier to localize the direction of sound. The brain uses loudness and timing differences between the sounds from each ear to determine where sounds are coming from. With only one hearing aid, these cues may not be available.

Subtle loudness and timing differences as sounds reach each ear also play a role in the understanding of speech in backgrounds of noise. The brain compares the information coming from both ears. Comparing these loudness and timing cues allows a person to better focus on some sounds while ignoring others. This is especially important for understanding one individual when there are many people talking.

Wearing only one hearing aid can be problematic for understanding speech coming from the unaided side. The person's head is in the way of the aided ear. Some of the sound will go around the head to reach the hearing aid, but many of the softer consonant sounds such as *th* or *f* may be lost. Although turning to face the speaker could overcome this loss in sound, this is not always practical when there are many people speaking.

Two hearing aids may also be perceived as more satisfactory than one because the amount of amplification needed in each ear is not quite as great when a person wears two hearing aids. The result is that a person is more likely to hear comfortably with two hearing aids. If a single hearing aid is worn, it may need to be set to an uncomfortably loud level to allow a person to hear well.

There is an additional medical reason why two hearing aids are preferable to one. Wearing only a single hearing aid can cause auditory deprivation in the unaided ear. After months or years of more sound stimulation to one ear than the other, the word understanding in the unaided ear may drop. Although the hearing level does not change, the clarity can. While an unaided ear may start out as being of some help to a person who begins by wearing only one hearing aid, it may be of less and less help over time. Wearing two hearing aids can prevent this. Some audiologists and hearing instrument specialists require their patients who want only one hearing aid to sign a waiver stating that they were informed of this possible consequence.

Although two hearing aids are usually best, there are valid reasons why a person might wear only one. The most obvious case would be a person with a hearing loss in only one ear. Similarly, a person with different severities of hearing loss in each ear might choose to wear a hearing aid in only the "better" ear. There are also a few people who, after trying two hearing aids, decide that they really prefer to wear only one. For these people, buying a second hearing aid makes little sense if they are sure that they will not wear it. The most common reason for wearing just one hearing aid, however, is cost. Many insurance plans do not include hearing aids as a covered benefit, leaving this expense to be paid directly out of pocket. Most people realize they would do better with two hearing aids, but this double expense is beyond the budget of some. They buy one and do the best they can with what they can afford.

Why bother if it won't give me perfect hearing?
Hearing is not an all-or-nothing sense. A person can have a small amount of hearing loss that does not functionally impact his or her everyday activities. From an individual's perspective, hearing loss only becomes an issue when it reaches the point when he or she can no longer hear what is necessary or desired. The goal in wearing hearing aids is not to restore perfect hearing but rather to prevent or minimize the functional impact of the hearing loss so a person can continue to pursue and enjoy the activities he or she considers necessary and important.

Hearing Aids and Health Concerns

Don't hearing aids cause ear infections?
Folklore holds that hearing aids can cause ear infections. This is similar to the belief that going out without a scarf or sleeping with wet hair can make a person sick. It flies in the face of medical fact.

Hearing aid use does, however, have the potential to create a more favorable environment for bacteria to grow in the ear canal. The ear canal is already a nice dark warm place, and the sweat caused by a poorly ventilated aid only makes the situation worse. Bacteria could not ask for a more perfect environment. This is precisely why most hearing aid manufacturers put a small air vent through the hearing aid that prevents any buildup of moisture. If there is a known history of ear infections or drainage, the air vent is made a little larger to allow even more air into the ear.

While hearing aids do not cause ear infections, they can aggravate an existing ear infection. If there is a mild infection in the ear canal itself, the hearing aid can rub the bacteria on the surface of the ear canal deeper into the skin, making matters worse. If the ear swells from the infection, then the hearing aid can rub even more, causing greater irritation. This is one of the reasons that a medical examination is recommended prior to purchasing hearing aids. The examination can rule out potential problems such as an ear infection.

Wouldn't hearing aids keep my ears from draining?

Folklore is the likely source of this view, also, in that it holds that drainage is good because it lets the body rid itself of infection. The reality is contrary to this belief. There should not be drainage from a normal ear. Drainage is a sign of infection or disease that needs to be treated by a physician.

Don't hearing aids make people nervous?

The response to this statement is "sometimes yes"—at least initially. Most people with hearing loss had their hearing worsen slowly. Little by little they became used to a quieter world. They may reach a point where they find few sounds annoying or uncomfortable. Hearing aids can therefore cause quite a shock because they reintroduce "lost" sounds to the wearer. All of these sounds can be quite stressful, especially at first. As a person begins to become reacquainted with familiar sounds, however, he or she begins to adjust. The sounds become less annoying, and the nervousness passes. The only solution is time.

Actually, people who wear their hearing aids on a regular basis soon find they feel less nervous rather than more. Often people with untreated hearing loss fear they will misunderstand and appear foolish at home or at work. They can do their best but still get things wrong or respond inappropriately. They are at the mercy of their hearing loss. By making it possible for a person to hear better, hearing aids reduce the chance for error. A person can have increased confidence that he or she will be in control of the situation. Wearing hearing aids results in a person having less to be nervous about.

Wouldn't improving my hearing be at the expense of my vision?

There is the perception that when a person loses one of his or her senses, the other senses become sharper to compensate. The two most popular variations on this are that a blind person's hearing improves to compensate for his or her blindness or that a deaf person's vision improves to compensate for being deaf. The second of these variations sometimes serves as a concern about buying hearing aids. A person may believe that gaining hearing will decrease his or her vision.

People who evaluate vision and hearing will attest to the fact that a person's vision or hearing does not change with the loss of the other sense. What changes is how the person makes use of the remaining sense. A hearing-impaired person will watch more intently everything that is going on around him or her. A blind person will listen more intently. A person gets more out of the remaining sense because it is used more frequently and with more concentration. The acuity of the remaining sense, however, does not change.

After wearing hearing aids for a time, people may notice that they do not use their vision the way they used to. It is not, however, that people cannot use their vision as they did before. They do not have to use their vision in the same way. Rather than watching, the wearer of hearing aids can listen instead.

Wouldn't I become dependent on hearing aids?

Hearing aids are scary things because they indicate dependency. The process is sometimes viewed as a one-way street into disability and decline. People with this concern believe that once they put on a set of hearing aids, they will no longer be able to hear as well without them. For them, wearing hearing aids represents a transformation from a self-sufficient person into a disabled one. The situation can be compared to the fear of an alcoholic relapsing after taking just one drink. A person may feel some things are better not to start and that hearing aids are one of these.

The misconception in the above statement is that hearing aids are the object of dependence. Hearing aids are a tool that can help a person compensate for a hearing loss, but it is the sense of hearing itself upon which he or she is dependent. Hearing is essential in a world that relies on spoken communication. People depend on their hearing from earliest childhood to learn language, get an education, make friends, and earn a living. The realization that takes place after trying hearing aids is just how much had been missed before. A person wears hearing aids because they make it possible to hear better and to participate more fully in a hearing world.

This issue of perceived dependence is exacerbated by other problems associated with aging and can be depressing. People may find their visual acuity declining. They may find the number of their health problems increasing. They recognize that they are slowing down in general. Now they find that their hearing is worsening and they need hearing aids to hear.

People are generally more willing to accept the idea of wearing eyeglasses or contact lenses to compensate for a vision problem than they are to accept hearing aids to compensate for a hearing loss. With eyeglasses, there is seldom a perception of decline, worry about dependence, or perceived stigma of being handicapped. Impaired vision is recognized as the problem and eyeglasses or contact lenses are accepted as the treatment or cure. If only there was this kind of understanding and focus regarding hearing loss and hearing aids.

Couldn't using hearing aids make my hearing worse?

Hearing aids should not make a person's hearing worse. The goal of hearing aids is to boost sounds up to a level that a person can hear without making the sounds uncomfortably loud. By limiting the maximum hearing aid output, the volume is kept within a safe range. This is not to say that some loud sounds will not be annoying. Important sounds like police and fire sirens need to be loud to draw a person's attention immediately.

Even though hearing aids do not make a person's hearing worse, people sometimes have the perception that their hearing gets worse after wearing them. What happens is that as people wear their hearing aids they get used to hearing better and more easily. They get used to a world full of sound. When they take the hearing aids off, they are more aware of what they cannot hear. Their hearing has not changed, but their expectation to hear has.

The few people with very severe or profound hearing losses may be an exception to the above statement. If a person's hearing is so bad that he or she hears nothing until the sound reaches a potentially damaging volume, then it is impossible for a hearing aid to help without the possibility of it causing harm. This person has a choice. He or she can go without hearing aids in an attempt to preserve their remaining hearing. This low-risk strategy offers a low reward: the patient remains functionally deaf. The alternative is to be able to hear with hearing aids, but with no guarantee for how long. Most people in this situation choose hearing aids because the small amount of hearing they do have is already of no use without them. They feel they have a lot to gain and very little to risk.

Don't hearing aids cause tinnitus?

Tinnitus is a perceived ringing, roaring, or cricket-like sound that is not actually present in the outside world. At a minimum it can be a nuisance; in a more extreme form it can cause lack of sleep or depression and has even been associated with suicide. People who have tinnitus worry about doing anything to their ears for fear it could make their tinnitus worse. People who do not have tinnitus worry they may get it. This concern can sometimes cause people to avoid hearing aids.

Tinnitus is not caused by hearing aids. The most common cause of tinnitus is nerve damage. Nerve damage also results in hearing loss that prevents outside sounds from covering up (masking) the tinnitus.

Rather than making tinnitus worse, hearing aids can serve to mask it. By bringing in outside sounds, hearing aids help people hear what is going on around them instead of what is going on inside them. Hearing aids do not cure tinnitus, but for many people with hearing loss, they can effectively mask it.

Wearing hearing aids can have one other beneficial side effect for people with tinnitus. There is a phenomenon known as residual inhibition in which the masking effect of the hearing aids seems to carry on for a short while after the hearing aids are removed. The reason this occurs is unknown, but the end result is that a person has an increased chance of falling asleep before their tinnitus reoccurs.

Won't hearing aids make me dizzy?

The inner ear controls both hearing and balance. Some people therefore fear that any change to their hearing might also affect their balance. This can be a real concern if the intervention under consideration is an invasive ear surgery that might damage the balance portion of the inner ear. The use of hearing aids, however, does not involve this kind of invasive procedure. The concern that the amplified sound of a hearing aid would produce dizziness is also unlikely to be realized unless there is something dramatically wrong with the ear. An easy way to test this fear is to turn the volume of a television to a high setting. If the loud sounds from the television do not cause dizziness, then the amplified sound from a hearing aid will not either.

Hearing Aids and Comfort

Won't hearing aids make my ears hurt?

When fitted correctly, hearing aids should not hurt. Pain is a signal that something is wrong. Custom-fit hearing aids will generally feel better in the ears than mass-manufactured ones, but even these should not be uncomfortable. The whole process of custom fitting hearing aids is designed to result in a comfortable fit. When a hearing aid is made, the fitter places a soft foam or cotton plug deep in the ear canal and then squirts in a silicon solution that quickly hardens. This cast is pulled out of the ear (along with the plug) and serves as the template for the size and shape of the hearing aid. The fitter sends this cast along with the circuitry specifications to a hearing aid manufacturer who makes the hearing aid to fit the person's ear and hearing loss. An aid that is custom made in this way should fit the ear exactly and be very comfortable. If for some reason the fit is off slightly, the hearing aid fitter can grind and then buff the hearing aid until it does fit comfortably. Custom-fit hearing aids are expensive, but the benefit of this personalized process is unmatched comfort.

This is one of the main reasons that almost all hearing aids are custom fit.

Of course, not everyone can afford to purchase custom-fit hearing aids. Mail-order, used, or donated hearing aids may be more financially feasible options, and unfortunately these do not fit as well. People who report discomfort are usually wearing hearing aids that came from one of these three sources. It is easy to understand why a mail-order hearing aid made to some "average" ear canal size might not fit an individual's ear comfortably. Fortunately mail-order hearing aids are required to come with a money-back guarantee that allows their return if they are dissatisfactory or uncomfortable. It is also easy to understand why an aid made for someone else would not fit well. Although it may be uncomfortable, a used or donated hearing aid may be the only solution for those who cannot afford to purchase a new one. Fortunately, it is often possible to recase the hearing aid by removing the circuitry and putting it into a better-fitting shell. There is some cost to this, but it is much less expensive than a new hearing aid. The result should be a comfortable and well-fitting hearing aid.

Doesn't a hearing aid feel like a foreign body in the ear?

Although it takes time to get used to the feel of wearing a hearing aid, it becomes second nature after a while. Getting used to the feel of a hearing aid is not really different from getting used to the feel of wearing eyeglasses or earrings. Given time, wearing a hearing aid may seem no more foreign than wearing a hat.

Won't they block my ears?

Some candidates for hearing aids worry that wearing hearing aids will make their ears feel blocked or plugged. People who wear earplugs when they swim or work voice this concern most frequently. The earplugs block outside sounds and make it seem like their ears are plugged up and not working properly. Insertion of earplugs may also produce a slight pressure imbalance between the middle ear and the ear canal that can additionally make the ears seem blocked. Because hearing aids are worn in the ears much like earplugs, many worry that they will have this same side effect.

What has to be kept in mind is that, while both fit into the ears, hearing aids and earplugs are not the same thing. While earplugs muffle sound, hearing aids increase volume. Furthermore, hearing aids usually have an air vent that will not allow pressure to build up in the ear canal as can happen with earplugs.

Couldn't I be allergic to hearing aids?

A not uncommon misconception is that a person will buy hearing aids and discover that he or she is allergic to the material they are made from. If people can be allergic to latex and other relatively benign substances, why not the plastic used in hearing aids? A few people may even have known someone who reported being allergic to hearing aids. The person's ear may have itched or become sore or swollen after wearing a hearing aid. What else could it be but an allergy?

The majority of reported allergic reactions to hearing aids are not really allergies at all. One of the most common causes is an ill-fitting hearing aid that rubs a sore spot into the ear canal. The problem can begin when a person gets his or her hearing aids and become worse the more the aids are worn. It is easy to distinguish from an allergy because only the portion of the ear that is being rubbed is aggravated. The remainder of the ear that is in contact with the hearing aid shows no reaction. Simply grinding, buffing, or remaking the case of the hearing aid to improve the fit will solve the problem.

True allergic reactions to hearing aids are extremely rare. The average audiologist or hearing instrument specialist might only see a few cases in his or her entire career. If, however, the reaction is in fact due to an allergy, there are special hypoallergenic hearing aid materials that can be used so that even these people can wear hearing aids.

In Summary

The human ear is a marvelous structure in terms of complexity and sensitivity. Unfortunately, it is not impervious to the ravages of age, loud noise, infection, and disease. These and other agents produce physical damage that results in hearing loss. Fortunately, hearing aid use is an effective way to compensate for these hearing losses. Although hearing aids do not restore normal hearing, they allow a person to hear better, thus eliminating many of the functional limitations that make hearing loss so problematic. Hearing aids are comfortable to wear and will not damage a person's remaining hearing or overall health. Regrettably, the failure of people to recognize and accept the presence of hearing loss often precludes any benefit from this understanding.

2 Denial and Acceptance of Hearing Loss

Celia Roberts had been referred to my office for a complete hearing evaluation after failing a hearing screening performed by her primary-care physician. Mrs. Roberts did not feel she had a hearing problem. She acknowledged that she occasionally had trouble understanding people, but attributed the cause of the difficulty to others. Their speech was either too soft or indistinct.

A more complete history revealed that a hearing instrument specialist had informed Mrs. Roberts of the hearing loss years previously during a free test. He had recommended hearing aids. She had also been told of the loss following several hearing tests that had been performed as part of her employer's hearing conservation program. She believed the hearing instrument specialist only wanted to sell hearing aids and discounted what he had said. She felt the hearing tests performed where she worked were not accurate. Furthermore, she would not have come for our evaluation, but her husband had insisted. He was not present during her office visit.

It was evident as Mrs. Roberts struggled to hear and understand my questions that she had a significant hearing problem. Testing only served to confirm what was obvious. Mrs. Roberts sat with both her arms and legs crossed as I discussed her hearing results and how she could benefit from hearing aids. I was no more successful at convincing Mrs. Roberts that she had a hearing loss than those who had gone before. She was in denial.

Hearing loss can be traumatic and cause feelings akin to grief and loss. Denial is often a first line of defense against these feelings. In the book *On Death and Dying*, Elisabeth Kubler-Ross (1969) described five steps people go through when faced with the prospect of dying. These steps are denial, anger, bargaining, depression, and acceptance. People must work through each of the first four steps before they can come to acceptance. In the years following the book's publication, the value of this construct for understanding how people deal with death has gained wide recognition. The steps also began to be applied successfully to other situations involving grief, disappointment, or loss.

The above construct applies in the case of a hearing problem because there is the loss of a sense. As in dealing with death, the initial response to hearing loss is usually denial. A person may feel that he or she is fine and the problem rests with others mumbling or not speaking clearly. Anger may follow. The anger may be aimed at what the person sees as the cause of his or her hearing problem (a loud work environment, an accident, a medication, aging, and so forth) or it may be aimed at the situation in general. Displacement frequently occurs and the anger can be misdirected toward friends and family. Bargaining comes next, as a person attempts to postpone accepting or dealing with the hearing loss. This may manifest itself as a person saying he or she would do fine if only the television were turned louder. It might instead involve some kind of deal in which family or friends repeat what is said or go out of their way to make it easier for the person to hear. Depression may follow once a person begins to recognize all the ways the hearing loss affects and limits his or her life. A kind of hopelessness may result that can prevent or delay a person's considering the options he or she has for coping with the hearing loss. A person has to pass through these steps and come to accept the hearing loss before he or she can effectively deal with it. The steps may occur in the linear manner described or they may occur simultaneously. The process is rarely as neat and orderly as a person with hearing loss or his or her family and friends would wish.

This chapter describes the ways in which people express their denial of a hearing loss. These expressions of denial frequently include anger, avoidance, and bargaining. These feelings may be familiar to you. Maybe you have felt them yourself or know someone who has.

Denial

I don't have a hearing loss. It is only earwax.
A comforting belief for people with hearing difficulties is to think that earwax is the problem and not their hearing. They can completely control this situation. If they do not consider the earwax a problem, they could leave it alone. If they find it to be an aggravation, they can have their ears cleaned. The wax would not represent a permanent hearing loss, an ear disease, or anything frightening. All they would need is a quick cleaning and the hearing would be great. Believing that the problem is only earwax allows the person to feel comfortable in delaying any kind of medical or hearing evaluation or treatment. Furthermore, as long as they do delay, they can continue to believe the problem is wax.

Unfortunately, the majority of hearing losses are not caused by earwax. This is not to say that earwax cannot block sounds and cause hearing difficulties. If the hearing problem really were due to earwax, however, a person would be able to use an over-the-counter ear wash or have the wax removed by a doctor. Both of these options are cheap, effective, and readily available. Knowing that these solutions are available, a person would not spend years complaining that their problem was only earwax.

Everyone mumbles. If people would "talk plain" I wouldn't have a problem.
There appears to be a conspiracy influencing the way some individuals speak. To many people with hearing loss it seems that nearly everyone mumbles, speaks soft, talks fast, or runs their words together. They do not "talk plain" like everyone used to. Many people also feel this to be true on television and in the movies. While I have not personally witnessed this conspiracy, I have at least a couple of patients every week insisting that it is true. These people remember back when people did "talk plain" so they know for sure that this is not the way things are now.

One patient will blame the schools for not having taught people to use proper diction. Another will feel that people are lazy and cannot be bothered to speak correctly. There are still others who feel that people speak this way on purpose.

A person could choose to believe that there is a conspiracy of mumblers responsible for the reported hearing difficulties of many, but the more likely explanation is a hearing loss that is undetected or denied. The majority of hearing losses happen gradually. There is no noticed change because every day a person seems to hear like the day before. You may still understand those who speak loudly so a logical assumption might be to conclude that the people who are not understood do not speak clearly. The other logical but dismissed possibility, of course, is hearing loss. Diagnosis of and education about the hearing loss are the keys to helping people who are unaware they have a hearing problem. They usually find this explanation much more reasonable than a conspiracy of mumblers.

For someone still in denial even after the diagnosis of hearing loss, the story is a little different. These people are likely to continue to blame those persons around them for their hearing difficulties. They embrace the idea of a conspiracy of mumblers and see the people around them as conspirators if not the ringleaders. Friends and family who are not entirely alienated by this behavior can try to be helpful and supportive; it remains up to the person in question, however, to work through denial and to move beyond the conspiracy theory.

My hearing is not bad enough for me to need hearing aids.
A purist might argue that any amount of hearing loss, no matter how small, should be corrected. In contrast, some people claim that their hearing is not bad enough for hearing aids regardless of the severity of their loss.

Determining the point at which a person becomes ready for hearing aids is highly subjective. This is dictated as much by what a person wants or needs to hear as by his or her actual hearing level. There is no set amount of hearing loss at which everyone feels the need for hearing aids. If you hear well enough to understand the things you want, then you may not feel the need for hearing aids regardless of the actual amount of hearing loss. In contrast, you may want hearing aids to compensate for a very slight hearing loss if you want to hear well or have demanding hearing needs.

The above discussion assumes that you can recognize what is not being heard. Unfortunately, this is not always true given the nature of hearing loss. People with hearing loss know what they think they hear, but they are not always aware of what they did not hear or what was misheard. They may benefit from the help of an outside observer who can provide a different perspective. Family, friends, and coworkers can serve as the best source for this alternative view. These individuals are aware of whether the person hears or mishears. If their observations agree with the person's belief that he or she hears well enough, then hearing aids are not needed. If, however, their observations disagree with those of the listener, then it needs to be determined whether the person was simply unaware of the hearing loss or whether he or she is in denial.

How well I hear "beeps" doesn't really reflect my true hearing.

People sometimes assume that because they do not go around listening for beeping sounds in their everyday lives, the beeps they listen for during a routine hearing evaluation have no relevance for them. They may also feel that the quiet room in which the tests are performed does not represent any real-life condition. They are concerned about understanding people in everyday situations and do not think that the typical hearing tests provide any measure of this. How can a test performed with these contrived sounds be used to determine whether hearing aids are needed? Wouldn't testing with everyday sounds provide a much better measure of a person's hearing and of whether or not he or she is in need of hearing aids?

The initial part of a hearing evaluation involves listening for the softest sound that can be heard at a number of different pitches. The test is usually performed in a quiet "sound-proof" room. Beeps (tones) are used because the hearing sensitivity for any pitch can be measured in this way. The results can be compared from person to person and over time. A quiet room is used because the goal is to determine how the person hears under ideal circumstances. It is understood that a person will do worse when conditions are less ideal. But, a person cannot do better than in this ideal situation.

The idea of using real-world sounds to test hearing has a certain amount of appeal, but it is not usually very practical. The problem lies in everyone's real world being a little bit different. A person working in a mall has to hear different things and separate them out from a different noise background than a person driving a truck. Hearing at a football game presents different listening challenges than listening in a pub. Whose specific listening situations should be chosen as the basis for the hearing test?

The alternative to using real-world conditions is to test a person's hearing ability in the presence of some kind of standardized noise. Although hearing loss could be quantified in this way, the real value of this may instead be as a predictor of hearing aid satisfaction. The hypothesis is that people who retain the ability to distinguish speech from background noise will be more satisfied with hearing aids than those who cannot. Research is ongoing to find a standardized test that will allow hearing aid professionals to reliably calculate potential hearing aid benefit based on a person's discrimination of speech in noise.

In short, while testing a person's hearing with beeps may not closely resemble any real-world listening condition, it does provide an accurate and reproducible measure of a person's hearing under ideal conditions. It serves as a good starting point to determine if a person has a hearing loss and whether or not something needs to be done about it. All too often, however, a person in denial will use the argument that the hearing test does not represent a real-world condition to discount the hard evidence that there is a hearing loss.

My family doctor did not recommend hearing aids.

The role of a general practice physician is to look out for the overall health of their patients. There are a million things that can go wrong with the human body. A physician cannot test for every one of them every time he or she sees a patient. Physicians look for those problems that are most likely to occur and at those problems about which their patients complain. A physician's failure to recommend hearing aids to a person with hearing loss can often be an oversight rather than proof that there is no need. If the physician does not routinely test for hearing loss (and most do not), and if the patient does not mention a possible hearing problem, this oversight is likely. The only time that silence from a physician regarding the issue of hearing aids should be taken as proof that there is no need for them is when the hearing has actually been tested. Everything else is speculation and possibly denial.

My hearing is fine. Other people must have super hearing.

Out of all of the reasons and excuses for not wanting hearing aids, this one is my personal favorite. It is perhaps also the expression of denial that most accurately identifies someone with a hearing loss. Aside from the television studio of the *Bionic Woman*, no one talks about super hearing with the exception of people with hearing loss. Anyone who mentions super hearing probably has a hearing loss.

Rather than accepting that they might have a hearing loss, some people begin to attribute superpowers to friends or family members. Colorful tights and a cape may be optional, but their superpowers are perceived as real. A spouse can hear the doorbell ring, the microwave beep, the birds singing outside, and the pastor at church. A hearing-impaired person might instead tell of a son or daughter who can hear people in another room, the cat scratching at the door, or a toilet running upstairs. These people must obviously have super hearing to hear all of this. The worse an individual's hearing, the greater the tales of superpowers in others he or she tells.

The underlying mechanism responsible for all these tales of super hearing was described almost a century ago by Sigmund Freud. He described a defense mechanism called projection in which people shifted the perceived burden of their problem onto others. The application of this theory to hearing explains why it is sometimes easier for people to believe that others have superpowers than to believe that they themselves might have a hearing loss.

Anger

I don't want to wear hearing aids and you can't make me!

This is a classic example of someone expressing anger associated with hearing loss. This person is not ready to accept or deal with his or her hearing problem. Family and friends recognize the hearing loss and proactively encourage the person to address it. Unfortunately, their attempt at being helpful or supportive is often unwanted and can result in the above statement.

A friend or relative suggesting hearing aids can be seen as very intrusive. Hearing loss is often viewed as a personal health problem that is not anyone else's business. This suggestion can be viewed as even more offensive if it is construed as a controlling act. The most frequent example of this occurs when a son or daughter recommends hearing aids to a parent. After years of telling a son or daughter what he or she should and should not do, a parent is unlikely to be pleased about a possible reversal of roles. The parent may view his or her autonomy as being in jeopardy.

Friends and family of a person with hearing loss should recognize that they can provide information and be supportive while a person goes through the process of coming to accept his or her hearing loss. It is not possible, however, to force a loved one to successfully deal with hearing loss or wear hearing aids until he or she is ready. The hearing-impaired person should recognize that his or her friends and family are trying to be supportive and that they should not be the target of the anger and frustration that the hearing loss produces.

I don't need any more extra parts.
People can be understandably angry and frustrated when they must use assistive or prosthetic devices to compensate for health problems. This anger and frustration can also extend to hearing aids.

As people get older, it is frequently necessary to replace failed body parts or to compensate for those that no longer work well. While some of these replacements like a pacemaker or an artificial hip are effectively permanent, others like dentures, eyeglasses, canes, and walkers need to be used (and remembered) daily. All of these parts can be viewed as an unwanted reminder of decline or disability. These daily parts can additionally be viewed as a nuisance.

Hearing aids fall into the category of parts that require daily maintenance. It is necessary to put them on, take them off, clean them, and change batteries. Once a hearing loss reaches a certain level of severity, hearing aids are not really optional equipment if a person wishes to hear. In a person's anger and frustration, however, it is not unusual for him or her to declare hearing aids to be one part too many.

Bargaining and Avoidance

I will learn to lip-read.

Lip reading is a wonderful help to people with hearing loss. Much that might go unheard or that might not be heard clearly can still be understood with the help of a few visual cues. One quick look at a spouse can help a person to discern whether it was a "cat" or a "rat" that was exclaimed to be in the yard. The person may not have heard the first consonant sound but it does not matter with lip reading because a *c* looks very different from an *r*. When a *c* is spoken the lips are pulled back. With an *r* the lips are pushed forward and rounded. Had it been a "bat" that was seen, then the speaker's lips would have been pushed together for the *b*. Even though the first letter was not heard, you can still figure out what the speaker said.

But this strategy won't work for everything. Not all sounds are as visually distinctive as *b*, *c*, and *r*. You would be at a loss to determine whether the speaker had said "pat" or "mat." Try it yourself by saying each of these words in front of a mirror. They will be visually indistinguishable.

Understanding with lip reading alone would be difficult even if all of the spoken speech sounds were visually different. Imagine trying to watch the lips of a person with a large beard or a long mustache. Who knows what might be taking place under all that hair? Others may hide what they say by turning away, eating, or talking with a hand in front of their mouth. In real life the lip movements are not always visible. Lip reading is a great help, but it is not an alternative to hearing. In order to understand spoken language, a person still needs to hear.

All I have to do to hear better is cup my hand behind my ear.

A not uncommon observation is that it is easier to hear when you cup a hand behind your ear. This directs additional sound into the ear that would otherwise pass by. It is the physiologic equivalent of the ear trumpets, the original hearing aid that helped people years ago to hear by collecting additional sound. Occasionally, a person sees this as a preferable alternative to hearing aids. For very mild hearing loss, this strategy might be sufficient. All that would be needed is for the person to hold a hand up behind his or her ear whenever someone was talking. For anyone with more than a mild hearing loss or without the stamina to constantly maintain this position, however, hearing aids are a more practical option. Hearing aids would certainly be the more aesthetically pleasing choice!

Although a number of people suggest that they could cup a hand behind their ear to hear better, few actually intend to do so. The real intent is to use this as an excuse to avoid hearing aids.

I can turn up the television and do just fine.

If it is necessary to turn the television up loud to hear it well, then hearing in other situations is likely to be a problem also. Listening to the television is about as easy as hearing gets. The sound is clear, loud, and coming directly at the listener. Furthermore, most of the time you can see the person talking, so lip reading is possible. In the real world, on the other hand, sounds are often soft, unclear, directed elsewhere, or partially covered by other sounds. Even a slight hearing loss can make it difficult to hear. A person who can hear the television only when it is loud and clear is generally not going to do "just fine" in other more difficult situations without some kind of help.

If television is all that you care to hear, then you may indeed be able to get by. If a person lives alone, rarely goes out, has few relatives or visitors, and prefers to spend his or her day watching television, then turning up the television is all he or she may need to do. Neighbors who live nearby, however, may not consider this the best solution. Furthermore, if a person does wish to hear something other than the television, such as friends or relatives, they too will need to be turned up louder. Turning up the television will not do this.

I won't die if I don't get hearing aids.

The above statement sounds like the rationale used by some insurance companies to explain why hearing aids are not a covered benefit on their major medical policies. In rare instances a person may be run over by an unheard car, truck, or train, but under normal circumstances failing to hear is not usually fatal. Consider, for example, congenitally deaf persons who communicate through sign language. The majority of these individuals live full and happy lives as members of the deaf community. They do not miss the hearing they never had and their use of sign language prevents social isolation.

The situation for people who develop hearing loss, however, is different from those who were born deaf. People who have heard for a lifetime miss being able to hear. They may not die if they do not get hearing aids, but they should probably wear them if they want to maintain the same quality of life.

People with a history of hearing will also be dependent on spoken language to communicate. Unless they choose to learn sign language, they will be isolated. Their real choice is not between getting or not getting hearing aids. The choices are to continue to communicate with spoken language, to learn to communicate through sign language, or to become isolated. Although hearing aids are required for the first choice, few other life changes are needed. The other options require big changes. Learning sign language also has implications for friends and family as well as for the person who is hearing impaired. Learning it in isolation is a bit like being the only person in a community with a phone. You cannot make or receive calls. The third option is to give up and withdraw. Given these options, hearing aids start looking better.

I don't have to hear.

This is similar to the earlier statement, "I won't die if I don't get a hearing aid." Although the focus of each statement is on hearing aids, the underlying issue is communication. Just explained was that people in the deaf community can and do live full, happy, and productive lives without hearing. They do this, however, by communicating. Someone who thinks that hearing is unnecessary should ask himself or herself how it will be possible to communicate with others if these others cannot be heard.

There is a question that needs to be asked when a person says, "I don't have to hear" or "I won't die if I don't get hearing aids." The question is, why does the person no longer consider communication to be important? This attitude can represent a deeper problem. It may reflect family struggles, identity problems following retirement, depression, or a number of other problems. The person's biggest problem may not be a matter of hearing or not hearing.

I have too many other medical problems right now.
It is common for people with serious or chronic medical problems to choose to put off getting hearing aids. When prioritizing their care, they often wish to take care of their medical problems so they can maintain or regain their health. Even so, they often find that they can better take care of their primary concern if they are able to hear. Being able to hear lets them respond appropriately to their doctor's questions and lets them better understand the instructions that their doctor gives. Furthermore, being able to hear friends and loved ones can make it easier during this stressful time.

The choice to delay the purchase of hearing aids in the midst of medical problems can be involuntary. The combination of lost wages and medical bills can make the purchase of hearing aids a near impossibility. If a person does put off getting hearing aids as a result of medical prioritizing or financial realities, this should not be used as a denial of the importance of hearing. The hearing-impaired person should instead try to plan for the time when the hearing problem can be addressed.

People would expect me to attend more functions and be involved in more activities if I could hear better.
A person may use his or her inability to hear to get out of doing things. In this form of bargaining a person trades the possibility of being able to hear better with hearing aids for other rewards. He or she might use hearing loss as an excuse not to attend a son or daughter's school conference, claiming he or she would not be able to understand the teacher. A person might claim that he or she would love to be able to attend a spouse's class reunion; unfortunately, the person would be out of place since he or she would not be able to hear. One can picture all of the things a person would rather not have to do and then imagine how hearing loss might be used to get out of

doing some of them. For a person who is manipulative, this is good stuff!

To be successful at not doing things, it is usually necessary to be able to find someone else who will do them. Those who are manipulative discover that a hearing loss can also be helpful here. All that needs to be done is to shame other people into feeling that they are forcing someone with a handicap to do things that they themselves could easily do. When a master of manipulation has thrown love or friendship into this mix, there is little chance that he or she will not get what is wanted. The only way for someone else to have a chance to win this game is to not play. People need to recognize if someone is playing this game with them and make sure that they are not unknowingly playing it with others.

I can't wear hearing aids at the factory.

It is true that people who work in loud factories or in other extremely noisy vocations may not be able to wear hearing aids on the job. The goal in these settings is to try to block or reduce the volume of surrounding sounds so that the noise is not loud enough to damage a person's hearing. Earplugs or earmuffs are usually required in these places to prevent hearing damage. Routine testing is performed to be sure that hearing is in fact being protected. You definitely would not want to wear hearing aids to make the factory sounds louder. You would also not want to wear hearing aids under a set of earmuffs. This would negate the whole purpose of the earmuffs. Since workers usually speak loud or sometimes yell to overcome the factory noise, hearing aids are unlikely to be needed in this setting even if they could be worn.

The problem with using the above statement as a reason for not buying hearing aids is that the average person does not live his or her whole life in a factory. There are times a person might want to hear what is going on outside. Just because there may be occasional instances where hearing aids cannot be worn does not mean that they will not be beneficial the rest of the time.

I can't wear hearing aids while I exercise.

This statement, like the one above, is a legitimate concern that is sometimes applied inappropriately. In each case, a person has found one situation where hearing aids may not be practical for him or her and then conclude that this negates their value the rest of the time. It does not.

In fact, the blanket statement that hearing aids cannot be worn during exercise may itself be in error. The major concerns with exercise and hearing aids are that perspiration will damage the hearing aids or that they will fall out of the ears. Not all forms of exercise, however, cause a person to sweat excessively or are so high impact that a hearing aid would be dislodged. It is true that hearing aids might best be left out during a judo match or a professional wrestling bout, but if the exercise is walking, low-impact aerobics, or yoga, hearing aids may work well.

I swim a lot and can't wear hearing aids then.

Hearing aids are electronic devices that are not intended to get wet. Water shorts out the electrical components and causes the circuitry to corrode. Fortunately, swimming is not one of the activities where people frequently complain about listening difficulties. Even people who swim a lot find their greatest hearing problems to occur in other situations.

The argument that a person should not get hearing aids because he or she cannot wear them while swimming is another instance of a person taking a valid concern to an extreme. Similar arguments might also be made by people who scuba dive or mud wrestle. But, as was previously explained, having one situation where it may not be possible to use hearing aids does not deny their usefulness in other situations.

I am too old to use hearing aids.

Almost as common as younger persons saying they are not old enough for hearing aids are elderly persons saying that they are too old for hearing aids. The argument for being too old to wear hearing aids usually comes down to two bargaining points. People either feel they no longer need to hear or they do not think they will live much longer.

If a person is retired, lives alone, does not go out much, and feels that he or she usually hears well enough, why would this person want hearing aids? Knowing how to answer this question depends on whether the person really does hear well enough for his or her chosen lifestyle or whether the person has chosen a limited lifestyle because he or she cannot hear well enough to do otherwise. If the person does hear well enough for his or her lifestyle, then hearing aids may not be needed. If, however, the person has chosen to retire, stay home alone, or not pursue social activities because of the hearing loss, then hearing aids should be a serious consideration. Either way, this is not really a matter of age.

A related excuse for people avoiding hearing aids is the belief that they are very old and probably won't live much longer. The problem with this line of reasoning is in the fact that they are not now dead and do not know when they will be. Death might not occur for five, ten, twenty, or more years. Who knows? Why should someone suffer unnecessarily with hearing loss or let it limit his or her activities in whatever time is left?

The hearing aid center is too far away.

If you're resistant to getting hearing aids, the inconvenience of getting to a hearing aid center can be a useful excuse. For the elderly, disabled, or extremely rural person it may also be a valid concern. There are physically active people in good health, however, that also claim this as a reason for not getting hearing aids. They feel that their hearing loss is not as inconvenient as their having to travel across town.

While fitting under the umbrella of health care, selling hearing aids is also a business. People who are successful in business have to be willing to go to where their customers are. Although the era of managed care and HMOs has made it difficult for physicians to make house calls, many audiologists and hearing instrument specialists are more than willing to do so. If you can't get out to see a hearing aid professional, you can have the professional come to you.

Living in a small town or remote area where there is no hearing aid office can reinforce some people's belief that they would have to go too far to get hearing aids. This, however, is not always the case. The same rule applies here that business will go to where the customers are. A larger hearing aid practice may have branch offices in smaller towns that are staffed a few days per week or as needed. They may have an arrangement to use other local facilities. They may also be willing to drive from another town to make a house call. Living in a small town does not always prevent door-to-door vacuum cleaner salespeople from coming to one's house. It also may not prevent access to hearing aid professionals.

Elderly, disabled, or extremely rural people should not automatically assume that they would not have access to hearing aid services. These services are usually available if they investigate their options. But, if a person has access but stresses only the issue of inconvenience, this may be a case of avoidance.

Acceptance of Hearing Loss

Denial of a hearing loss is the first obstacle to better hearing. A person will not seek help for a problem he or she does not acknowledge. Even if the person recognizes the loss, he or she may not be ready or willing to deal with it. There may be anger, bargaining, avoidance, or depression, or a person may just be stubborn. The discussions in this chapter show how these reactions can prevent a person from being ready to consider hearing aids. A person must first accept his or her hearing loss and work through these issues. Family and friends can help this process along by being supportive and by providing information. They cannot, however, successfully force the issue. A frequent mistake is to try to focus on hearing aids before a person has truly accepted his or her hearing loss. Acceptance must come first.

Acceptance of hearing aids, however, does not automatically follow the acceptance of hearing loss. There are other obstacles to hearing aids, not the least of which are concerns about appearance or concerns that only masquerade as being about appearance. A person who fully accepts and appreciates his or her hearing problem can be stopped by these next obstacles.

3 Appearance and Deeper Concerns

Sandra Carson had come for an examination to discover if there was a medical or surgical solution for her hearing loss. A friend at her church had his hearing restored following middle ear surgery, and Sandra wondered whether this surgery might help her. Her examination and hearing test results showed her to have sensorineural hearing loss. It was explained that she had a different kind of hearing loss than her friend and that hers was not medically or surgically correctable. She was, however, an excellent candidate for hearing aids.

Although Mrs. Carson readily acknowledged her hearing loss and the difficulties it caused her as a librarian and a mother, she did not want hearing aids. She said that hearing aids were big and ugly and that she was not going to be seen wearing something like that. I explained that the way she wore her hair would hide any style of hearing aid. I additionally explained that she would be able to wear very small hearing aids that would not be noticeable even if she were to wear her hair up or pulled back. She still refused to consider hearing aids. The problem was not physical appearance.

Cosmetic objections are frequently given as a reason for not wanting hearing aids. A person may dislike the look of hearing aids or the way he or she looks while wearing them. A person might instead be more concerned that others would find the aids unsightly. The advertising for the smaller hearing aids can even reinforce the perception that a person should not be seen with them. One final group of concerns is that hearing aid use might affect a person's appearance in some unwanted or unforeseen way. All of these cosmetic issues can be obstacles to hearing aid use.

Greater obstacles, however, are often hidden beneath this façade of cosmetic concerns. The worry over appearance may mask feelings of shame or embarrassment. It may involve concerns about aging or weakness. It may cover feelings of helplessness or inadequacy. The existence of these underlying concerns was illustrated by the librarian's continued objections to hearing aids. She understood that no one else would see them. Still, she could not bring herself to wear them.

This chapter examines the cosmetic concerns that are the visible tip of this iceberg. More important, it also explores the underlying bulk of deeper concerns.

Cosmetic Concerns

The look of hearing aids.

A common perception is that no matter how hearing aids might be styled or how small they are made, they are ugly. This is an unfortunate perception because many of today's hearing aids are elegant in design. Years ago, most hearing aids were ugly. The available technology and materials required that they be large, made in unnatural colors, and lacking almost any form of aesthetics.

Hearing aid manufacturers today go to great lengths to make their hearing aids as cosmetically appealing as possible. The first of these efforts involves miniaturizing the aids until they can fit deep into the ear canal. If a person cannot see them, the way they look is not important. A completely-in-the-canal (CIC) aid is smaller than the tip of a finger and virtually invisible when in the ear (see fig. 3.1). This size hearing aid usually works well with the mild and moderate hearing impairments that account for the majority of hearing losses.

Larger, more visible hearing aids are likely to be needed with more severe hearing losses. This larger size does not mean, however, that the hearing aids must be unsightly. The fit, finish, and styling of hearing aids are much better than ever before. Today's hearing aids often have a lower profile than older hearing aids due to the miniaturization of electronics. This means that a new hearing aid may be thinner and not stick as far out of the ear.

In-the-ear hearing aids are usually made in beige, tan, light brown, and dark brown. The shades of these colors, however, can vary slightly among manufacturers. Hearing aid centers that sell multiple brands sometimes take advantage of this fact to select hear-

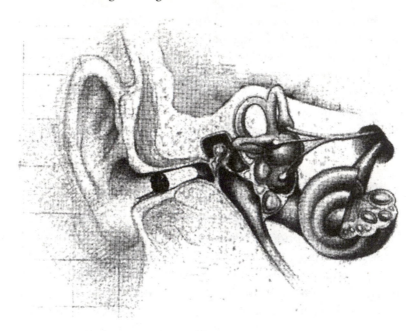

Figure 3.1. Cut-away view of a CIC hearing aid in the ear. Courtesy of Starkey Labs.

ing aids that will most closely match a person's skin tone. The larger behind-the-ear (BTE) hearing aids that tend to be everyone's greatest cosmetic concern come in a much wider array of colors. It is usually possible to find a BTE aid to match almost any skin color in the world's diverse population. Depending on personal preference, an aid could instead be colored to match a person's hair. This works exceptionally well when a person is wearing a hairstyle that covers the ears.

While today's hearing aids are not really ugly, they are often visible due to size or hairstyle. This is a reality that needs to be recognized. Being seen with hearing aids may be one of the costs of being able to hear.

The look of ears after hearing aids.
An infrequent concern regarding hearing aids and appearance is that the hearing aids will in some way affect the look of the ears

themselves. The first of these concerns is that the physical presence of a hearing aid in the ear will push against the ear, causing it to stick out away from the skull. This does not happen. The individualized fitting process ensures that the shape of a hearing aid will exactly match the shape of the ear. A hearing aid will not push the ear in any direction.

A second concern is that hearing aids will cause a person's ears to stretch out and become big. The people who have this fear most often know someone who has hearing aids. They have learned that if a person wears the same hearing aid for a number of years the ear will stretch slightly around it making the hearing aid fit loosely. Once this happens, the hearing aid is remade to be slightly larger or replaced with a new one that fits better. This process is repeated every few years as necessary. Taken to an extreme conclusion it is possible to understand how a person might envision this process eventually enlarging someone's ears.

Fortunately, this process of an ear stretching slightly around a hearing aid does not go to these extremes. The changes in the ear may be enough to allow the hearing aid to feel loose or for some of the sound from the hearing aid to leak out of the ear, but usually not enough to be visibly apparent. This is true even for people who have worn hearing aids for many years. The size and shape of a person's ears may change very slightly following years of hearing aid use, but Dumbo-shaped ears will hardly result.

A third concern is that hearing aid use may necessitate increased grooming of the ears. An unfortunate fact for many people is that as they grow older hair quits growing out of the top of their head and begins growing out of their ears. Like the belief that shaving causes a beard to grow faster, some people fear that wearing a hearing aid will somehow affect the hair in their ears. They may think that more hair will grow or that it will grow faster. Although I am aware of no scientific study dedicated to this subject, there does not appear to be any relation between hearing aid use and ear hair. Just as in the general population, some people who wear hearing aids have hair in their ears and some do not. Hearing aids do not make any difference.

There are other more obscure fears regarding how the appearance of the ears may be harmed by hearing aids. These fears are also unfounded. Hearing aid use does not affect the shape or appearance of the ear.

Deeper Concerns

Hearing loss as a private versus public matter.
It should come as no surprise that many people with hearing loss fear that wearing hearing aids will advertise their disability. Basically the issue is that the person feels an invasion of privacy. Hearing loss as a private versus public matter has already been mentioned in regard to family or friends suggesting hearing aids. This suggestion was viewed as an unwanted intrusion into a private affair. If people consider hearing aids an out-of-bounds subject for friends or family, it is likely to be an even more sensitive issue with strangers. Other health concerns are treated in confidentiality. There are laws that protect a person's medical privacy. If a person does not wish to share his or her medical problems, he or she does not have to. Someone suffering from heart disease, impotence, or mental illness would certainly not be required to advertise. Wearing hearing aids can sometimes be viewed in this context.

Many potential hearing aid users are reluctant to recognize that family, friends, acquaintances, and even strangers are usually well aware of the hearing loss. People do not have to see hearing aids to know that someone is hearing impaired. They know of the problem because the person is not understanding what is said or is not responding appropriately to what is said. Although hearing aids may be a visible indicator of a hearing loss, they can be less noticeable than not wearing hearing aids and pretending that a hearing loss does not exist.

Associations with aging.
It is a well-recognized fact that hearing tends to decline with age. The resulting perception is that hearing loss is a sign of aging. While the initial statement may be statistically true, it is not necessarily applicable when applied on an individual basis. Although the chance of needing hearing aids increases with age, some people will not

need hearing aids even if they live to be quite old. In fact, only about one-third of people sixty-five years of age or older have a hearing loss severe enough that they would benefit from hearing aids. The percentage of people needing hearing aids would be higher for eighty- or ninety-year-olds, but there would still be many in these groups with good hearing. We should not simply assume that because a person is old, he or she has a hearing loss and needs hearing aids. If a hearing loss is due to aging, however, a person should recognize that the purpose of hearing aids is to compensate the hearing loss, not to compensate for being old.

People are often surprised to learn that it is not just the elderly who can have a hearing loss. Young people can also have hearing problems. Many of the hearing losses for these younger individuals are medically or surgically correctable, but some are not. Young people with hearing losses that are not medically or surgically correctable must rely on hearing aids. They may include children who were born deaf or who developed a hearing loss shortly following birth. Also included in this not-old group would be children or adults with a hereditary hearing loss or a hearing loss caused by noise exposure, disease, trauma, and the like. It is very common for construction or factory workers, ambulance drivers, landscapers, and musicians to have hearing problems at a younger age due to excessive and loud noises in their professions. These people are unlikely to consider themselves to be old simply because they have a hearing loss. They may, however, fear that others will consider them to be old. This serves as the underlying basis for many objections regarding the appearance of hearing aids. As long as hearing aids can be seen, there is the very real risk of this association.

Sexuality.

Concerns about sexuality can also underlie cosmetic objections to hearing aids. A woman may not be able to view herself as beautiful or alluring if she were to wear them. A man may worry about how others view his masculinity or virility. Even if secure in their own sexuality, both men and women may worry about the conclusions that might be drawn by others. The previously mentioned associations between hearing loss and age complicate these matters. Our society associates youth with beauty. Hearing aids are often associated with old age, which is in turn associated with declining beauty.

These concerns can surface in many forms. Samuel Toth was a forty-eight-year-old construction worker who feared that hearing aids might lead to his divorce. His underlying belief was that his younger wife might no longer view him as attractive or virile. His wife felt that the greatest risk to their marriage was from the loss of communication the hearing loss caused. This was what she found unattractive. After much discussion, he agreed to try hearing aids. He heard better, and the couple did not divorce.

Fortunately, Mrs. Toth was right in that it is the ability to share things with a spouse that usually brings and keeps couples together. Wearing hearing aids makes it easier to do this. Hearing aids usually decrease, not increase, marital stress. This is especially true if the hearing-impaired spouse has been in denial.

Jeremy Stanton was another person who had concerns about hearing aids and sexuality that were associated with age. Rather than preventing him from trying hearing aids, however, his concerns caused him to quit using hearing aids. Jeremy had been born with a hearing loss. He had successfully worn behind-the-ear hearing aids for the last fifteen of his sixteen years. Jeremy's parents brought him for a consultation because he had recently "lost" one set of hearing aids and refused to wear his new set. They also reported he had changed from an average student to a failing student. Jeremy was shy about voicing his feelings, but the major issue was that he did not feel that girls would find him attractive with his hearing aids. He wanted to date and believed that his hearing aids stood in the way. Happily, switching to smaller inconspicuous hearing aids resolved his issues. He was less self-conscious about wearing the smaller hearing aids, and he could once again hear in class. He could also hear the girls.

Concerns about the affect of hearing loss and hearing aids on sexuality can be extremely difficult to address. Sexuality can be another off-limits subject and combining it with the distasteful subject of hearing aids only makes it more so. A spouse or very close friend may be able to successfully broach this subject, but it can be extremely difficult for others. More often, the ability to communicate is traded for the perception of preserved sexuality.

Power, weakness, and hearing loss.
Hearing-impaired schoolteachers exemplify one interplay of power, weakness, and hearing loss. A teacher may fear that his or her students or other children in the school will become aware of the hearing loss and use it against him or her. The children may only pretend to talk in order to make fun of the teacher. The children may mock the teacher in other ways. This is a real concern because it is a threat to a teacher's authority. Many teachers with hearing loss reject hearing aids for this reason.

The sight of hearing aids, however, does not make a teacher the biggest target. It is all of the things he or she cannot hear or would mishear without them. For children this is a greater gold mine of opportunity to make fun than the use of hearing aids. Furthermore, a teacher can usually hide his or her hearing aids by wearing a small style or by changing his or her hairstyle. This greatly reduces the chance that students would even be aware of the hearing aids. Hiding an uncorrected hearing problem would be much more difficult.

The prospect of wearing hearing aids can also be viewed as a sign of weakness. A construction worker may be reluctant to admit that years of noise exposure have taken a toll on his or her hearing. To do so would be admitting weakness. This person may be even less likely to want to be seen with hearing aids because it would advertise not only the presence of a hearing loss, but also that the person cannot cope with the hearing loss without the help of hearing aids. Both the hearing loss and the need for hearing aids are indications of weakness. The person can either deny the hearing loss or overcome these emotional issues. All too often it is the former that happens. The person and his or her family are left to suffer the hearing loss.

A business executive with hearing loss may face different issues regarding power and weakness. The concerns here, however, might involve the loss of the ability to achieve, to advance, or to remain in charge. An advertising executive may fear that he or she would no longer be given the good accounts. An engineer may worry about not being considered for challenging projects. A junior vice president may fear that hearing aids could interfere with his or her chances for advancement to a more senior level. A person who has fought his or her way to the top may fear that subordinates might see the hearing loss as indicating vulnerability. In each of these instances, the person views hearing aids, more than the hearing loss, as a potential detriment.

Personal and private image.

One of the most difficult problems underlying cosmetic objections to hearing aids is when a person believes and internalizes all the stereotypical beliefs about hearing aids. If a person believes that hearing loss is associated only with old age, that hearing aids are ugly, that they negatively impact sexuality, that they will harm personal relationships, or that they will hinder job performance or the chance for advancement, he or she will have a difficult time accepting and dealing with his or her own hearing loss. All of this can create a devastating impact on a person's self-image. The person may feel shame, embarrassment, helplessness, inadequacy, or anxiety or become depressed. Is it any wonder that so many people instead choose denial?

The issue of image is not, however, only an internal problem. The expectations of how people should look in our youth-oriented society can be difficult when people with hearing loss have to present an "appropriate" public image. This concern could apply to almost anyone in the media. They have to present the image that people want to see. If they fail to do this, they may not be in the spotlight. Concerns about public image can also apply on an individual basis. If a person's goal is to appear young and invulnerable, hearing aids could be a problem.

There is a common image of hearing aids as representing handicap. This association is sometimes so strong that a person overlooks his or her own hearing loss as being the real problem. The perception is that a person does not have a handicap until he or she uses hearing aids. Webster's dictionary defines a handicap as "having a physical or mental disability that substantially limits activity especially in relation to employment or education." The focus of this definition is on function, not appearance. There is no question that hearing loss can be considered a handicap. Wearing hearing aids cannot. Hearing aids are the remedy. Recognizing this distinction can help to correct negative stereotypes that are internalized and the problems of self-image that can result.

What cannot be said enough is that the most visible signs of a hearing loss are the limitations it can produce. A small hearing aid deep in the ear canal or a large hearing aid covered by a person's hair is not going to be as obvious as misunderstanding or responding inappropriately to what is said. This is true even if the hearing aids are visible. A bank teller is not likely to notice a customer's hearing aids. He or she will notice being asked to repeat. Similarly, hearing aids are less likely to draw attention to a student in class than his or her not wearing them and frequently misunderstanding or doing poorly. The reduction in actual disability outweighs the visual impact of hearing aids.

The hope exists that a more realistic image of people with hearing loss will develop as the baby-boom generation ages. This would ideally erase many of the negative stereotypes associated with hearing aids. It might also present opportunities for people with an entrepreneurial spirit. Only one step behind the acceptance of hearing aids that are visible might be designer hearing aids. The big question for people with hearing loss might not be whether or not to get hearing aids, but rather, what fashion statement they wish to make with the ones they buy.

Final Thoughts on Hearing Aids and Appearance

Cosmetic objections are a real concern that can prevent people from using hearing aids. The hearing aid industry's response has been to make hearing aids smaller so that they are less visible. This strategy has had some success but there are still people who will object to even the tiniest ones. The reason this occurs is that there is usually more involved than only a superficial concern about appearance. There can be underlying concerns about privacy, aging, embarrassment, power, or sexuality. These and other issues can appear individually or in combinations. With a little introspection, a hearing-impaired person who objects to the appearance of hearing aids may find that his or her real concern is something deeper. Family and friends of a person with hearing loss need to be aware that an objection to appearance is not necessarily going to be overcome by a small hearing aid or a change in hairstyle.

4   Fears and Doubts

A person may be psychologically ready to try hearing aids but reluctant to do so. This is often the result of unresolved fears or concerns. Some of these stem from a lack of information, or more often, from misinformation about hearing aids themselves. The concerns fall into four general categories. The first involves concerns about hearing aid performance. This includes the worries that hearing aids might not work, that they would only make things louder, or that they might have poor fidelity. Maintenance issues comprise the second category. A couple of the issues in this category would include concerns such as "I don't know how to take care of them" or "they might be too complex for me to work." The third category involves concerns about getting used to hearing aids. This could involve getting used to the feel of hearing aids, the way they sound, or simply the habit of using them. The final category involves unexpected fears and phobias about hearing aids. This chapter addresses these concerns and misunderstandings.

Performance

Burt Evans was seventy-two years old when I first saw him as a patient. He reported a hearing loss of several years' duration that had gradually worsened. Understanding his wife, daughter, and grandchildren had become increasingly difficult. He reported hearing well on the telephone and when listening to the television. His wife, however, said the television was intolerably loud and that he sometimes misunderstood strangers on the phone. Although he had retired from the police force seven years before, he still got together with the "guys" for golf and poker. He was also having trouble hearing when with them. Mr. Evans recognized that he needed help to hear better, but he was resistant to hearing aids. His mother had worn a hearing aid twenty years before but had had no appreciable increase in her ability to hear. Mr. Evans feared that he would do no better. He did not recognize that the performance of hearing aids had improved since then.

This is only one example of how a person who was ready for hearing aids could be sidetracked by concerns about performance. Below are other concerns that often produce this same result.

I thought hearing aids didn't work.

One of the most common concerns people have about hearing aids is that they may not work. There are three main reasons why people believe this. The first reason is related to the actual limitations of hearing aids. Second, if you are basing your attitudes on older hearing aids, much that once was true may no longer apply. Finally, the opinion that hearing aids do not work can come from personal experience.

Hearing aids do not restore normal hearing. They instead compensate for hearing loss. Hearing aids work by amplifying the volume of sounds a person cannot hear to a level that is audible. Even if this is done clearly and efficiently, the ear itself may still garble, distort, or fail to correctly process some sounds. People hear better with hearing aids, but the ears themselves do not always let them hear perfectly.

In addition to the listening difficulties that can result when an ear distorts the sound that a hearing aid provides, it can be difficult to make soft sounds loud enough for a hearing-impaired person to hear without making moderate and loud sounds uncomfortably loud. This limits how loud a hearing aid can be set. If the aid is turned up to a level that would be optimal to hear, it may seem too loud. If it is turned down to a level that is comfortable, the volume may not be optimal to hear. This was true of almost all of the older hearing aids and is partially responsible for the perception that hearing aids do not work.

A person who knows someone who wears hearing aids may also make the statement that "hearing aids don't work." The person observes that even with hearing aids, the user may not hear the softest sounds or occasionally misunderstands what is said. Based on this observation, he or she concludes that hearing aids do not help. If the person were to ask the opinion of the hearing aid user, however, the conclusion would likely be different. From the user's perspective, the hearing aids boost sound from a volume that is difficult or impossible to hear to a volume where he or she will have a much better chance of hearing and understanding. The person won't say that hearing aids are perfect, but he or she is likely to say that they are a great help.

A comparison could be made with the experiences of the character Steve Austin on the television show *The Six-Million-Dollar Man*. As you may recall, he was a pilot who had a near fatal airplane crash that left him missing an eye, an arm, and both legs. The scientists in the story were proud that they could rebuild him using bionic parts that made him stronger and faster than ever. He could run, jump, chase bad guys, and do all of the other things that people have come to expect during a prime-time adventure story. Did they work? Sure. But they also creaked when strained.

Don't hearing aids just make things louder?

Hearing aids do work by making things louder, but they do not "just" make things louder. They make sounds selectively louder. This is an important distinction because it directly impacts how well and how comfortably a person will be able to hear.

Early hearing aids selectively amplified sounds to give people help at the pitches where they had the majority of their hearing loss. The goal was to boost all of the pitches necessary to understand speech up to a volume that would be audible to the user. If a person had a high-pitched hearing loss, the hearing aids would amplify the higher frequencies. If the loss were low pitched, the lower frequencies would get the boost. What these early hearing aids could not do was recognize the loudness of incoming sounds. They provided a set amount of amplification regardless of input level. The result was that by the time the soft sounds were made loud enough to hear the loud sounds were made much too loud to be comfortable. Limiting the maximum output helped, but too many sounds still received more amplification than was needed or was comfortable.

Newer hearing aids can recognize the loudness of an incoming sound and increase the amplification as needed. A soft sound may be given a lot of boost to get it up to a level that will sound soft but be audible for the user. A moderately loud sound may only be given a small amount of boost to nudge it into the middle of a person's hearing range. A loud sound may be left alone or even reduced slightly if too loud. The goal is to take the full range of sound and compress it between the softest level a person can hear and the level that begins to become uncomfortably loud. This makes sounds not just audible, but audible at levels that are comfortable for an individual user.

Beyond simply looking at what pitches to amplify and how much to amplify them, a few of today's hearing aids can also select what kinds of sounds to amplify. Since the usual goal of wearing hearing aids is to be able to understand speech, the hearing aids are designed to emphasize speech sounds relative to non-speech sounds. The hearing aids can do this to some extent because speech is a dynamic stimulus changing in pattern, loudness, and frequency. Sounds that match the characteristics for speech are amplified while more steady state noises (assumed to be background noise) are not amplified or are amplified less. This is all much different from "just" making things louder.

I tried hearing aids years ago and they did not help.
On the surface, this is a very reasonable argument for not getting hearing aids. It is the "been there, done that" argument. What would be the point of trying hearing aids again if a person had already done this and the hearing aids were not helpful? There is a potential flaw, however, in this line of reasoning. The flaw is the underlying assumption that nothing has changed since hearing aids were tried.

The first thing that has likely changed is the hearing aid technology itself. If a person tried hearing aids only a few years ago, the hearing aids he or she tried were very different from those that are available today. The older hearing aids were analog devices. This is the same technology used in records, cassettes, and conventional television. Many of the newer hearing aids are digital devices that employ the technology used in compact discs (CDs), computers, and high-definition television. The difference is that analog devices process their signals as a voltage while digital devices process them as numbers. Although this might appear to be a subtle difference hardly worth mentioning, it is an important difference. Once a signal is coded as numbers, changing one or more of the numbers in the program can modify the signal in almost an infinite number of subtle or dramatic ways. In an analog device replacing some or all of the circuitry is the only way to make dramatic changes. Lesser changes could be made with a volume control, tone control, and so forth, but the degree of subtlety would not approach what could be achieved digitally. Adjusting hearing aids to compensate best for a person's individual hearing loss requires subtlety. The newer hearing aids have this subtlety. Many people who tried but did not like analog hearing aids in the past are now successful digital hearing aid users.

The second thing that may have changed since a person had tried hearing aids is the hearing itself. People often try hearing aids for the first time when their hearing loss reaches the point that it begins to cause listening difficulties. After initially trying hearing aids a person may conclude that he or she does not really need them yet. With time, however, a person can go from being in a position to benefit only occasionally from hearing aids to the point that normal conversational speech cannot be heard well without them. There would then be no question that hearing aids would help.

Shouldn't I wait before getting hearing aids since they keep getting better?

Hearing aids do keep getting better. The sound quality is better than ever before as are the aesthetics. With the continuing trends of hearing aids becoming smaller, less visible, clearer sounding, more comfortable, and easier to use, a person might be inclined to wait for the next one that might be even better. The problem is that this is a never-ending process. A person with hearing loss needs to hear now! This wait-and-see strategy does not solve the immediate problem. Years down the road when today's hearing aids are worn out, the replacement set can include any further advances.

Won't background noise keep me from hearing?

Some people fear that all they will hear with hearing aids is background noise. They worry that they will understand less with hearing aids than without them because of this noise. This is not, however, the case. There *is* more noise with hearing aids than without; however, some of this noise contains desired information. Unless people are speaking louder to make up for the hearing loss, the ratio of the speaker's volume to noise is no worse for a hearing-impaired person with hearing aids than for a normal-hearing person without hearing aids. What is different is that a person with hearing loss is less likely to be able to pick out what he or she would like to hear from within a background of noise than a person with normal hearing. This difference is not due to hearing aids, however; rather, it is the result of nerve damage.

I didn't think hearing aids could help on the phone.

Hearing on the telephone can be very difficult for a person with a significant hearing loss or poor word understanding. In everyday conversations many of these people will rely heavily, often more than they know, on lip reading to help them recognize the sounds they do not hear or do not hear well. On the phone they cannot do this. They must depend entirely on their hearing.

People with mild hearing losses generally do well on the phone even without a hearing aid because most telephones are fairly loud. The situation changes, however, with larger hearing losses. The average telephone is not loud enough for a person with a severe hearing loss. It is also a problem when a person hears fairly well at some but not all pitches. The phone will seem loud enough even though some speech sounds may be inaudible. The listener hears the person talking, but may not understand. In each of these cases a hearing aid can be helpful to make things loud enough to be heard while simultaneously balancing the pitches so that a person has a chance at hearing all of the different speech sounds. This does not mean that a person who wears hearing aids will hear perfectly on the phone, but he or she should at least hear better.

When people talk about not hearing well on a telephone, they are not usually talking about simply hearing what is said; instead, they are talking about understanding what is said. It is necessary to hear a conversation to have a chance to understand it, but just because it is heard does not mean that it will always be understood. A hearing aid can improve a person's chance of hearing on the phone, but it does not guarantee that the ear will process all of the sound correctly. This does not mean that hearing aids will not help, but hearing loss can limit the hearing aids' ability to solve the problem.

In some instances, nerve damage in the inner ear can cause the word understanding to be so poor that a phone is of little use even with a hearing aid. So little of what is heard is understood that, without the help of lip reading, it is nearly impossible to have a conversation. In these most extreme cases where a hearing aid is not helpful, a telephone device for the deaf (TDD) can be used. This is a special typewriter that plugs into the phone line. Rather than speaking into the phone and listening, the person types and reads. A person can carry on this kind of conversation with other people who have a TDD or with a special service that will verbally relay what is said to a hearing person using a normal phone. This equipment has been available for years and is in wider use than generally recognized. A hearing aid does work well for most people, however, limiting the need for this more extreme method of using the phone.

I tried a friend's hearing aid and it didn't help.

While the above statement can be very true, it is not necessarily relevant. If a hearing aid made for one person does not work for someone else, it does not necessarily mean that it does not work well for its owner or that a different appropriately fit hearing aid could not work well for this second person. It only means that this particular hearing aid did not work well for someone other than its intended user.

Hearing aids are custom made to compensate for an individual's particular hearing loss. The hearing loss might be low pitched or high pitched. The loss might be small or large. One person may tolerate loud sounds well, while another person may be very sensitive to loud sounds. Unless a person's hearing loss is exactly the same as someone else's loss, his or her aid will not appropriately compensate for the other person's hearing loss. The prescription will be wrong.

Most people cannot wear a friend's eyeglasses, either. While no one expects to be able to wear a friend's glasses, many people mistakenly expect hearing aids to be interchangeable.

The fit of a hearing aid is also specific to an individual. The size and shape of each person's ears are a little different. A hearing aid not made for the person may be so tight as to be uncomfortable or so loose that it falls out of the ear. Aside from the issue of comfort, an inappropriate fit can also allow sound to leak out of the ear. At a minimum, the person does not hear as well as he or she should because the sound does not stay in the ear where it belongs. This escaping sound can also cause the hearing aid to whistle.

If everyone had exactly the same hearing loss, the same size and shape of ears, and the same tolerance for different sounds, then trying a friend's hearing aid would make good sense. But since this isn't the case, trying a friend's hearing aid doesn't really count as a trial run.

I don't believe all the hype in the hearing aid commercials.
This can be true with commercials for most products, and hearing aids are no exception. The whole point of commercials is to sell a product. It is not necessarily to inform. Hearing aid advertising is not any more or less honest than advertising for other products. Sure, there is hype in some of the commercials for hearing aids, but this is an expected part of the world in which we live. It is not a reason to keep from hearing.

The best or most trustworthy hearing aid advertisements are successful hearing aid users. They will tell their family and friends how much the hearing aids help and the centers where they were purchased. This information spreads throughout a community by word of mouth. Physicians and other professionals refer to these centers because they have a good reputation. Trustworthy dealers may not necessarily need to advertise or they may advertise very little.

People do not have to believe hearing aid commercials. All they have to do is find a friend, a relative, or an acquaintance who is happy with their hearing aids and who feel they were treated fairly and professionally by their audiologist or hearing instrument specialist.

There are too many hearing aid choices. How do I know which one to buy?

With all of the hearing aid manufacturers proclaiming in newspaper, magazine, radio, and television advertisements that they make the best hearing aids, it is no wonder that you may be confused. You'll have to make choices about brands, sizes, and circuitry options. A hearing aid that might be made to appear the very best on television may not be at all appropriate for some hearing losses. Additionally, there is no readily available guide that people can use to match their hearing loss and listening needs to a specific hearing aid. The fear exists that a person may pay twice as much as he or she should for a hearing aid that is less than optimal for his or her hearing loss and listening needs.

The problem is not too many hearing aid choices. Instead, there is either too little information about these choices or too little help sorting through the information that is available. People often do not know where to look for information about hearing aids or are instead overwhelmed by the amount of information once they find it. They start accumulating pamphlets, brochures, and videotapes from various hearing aid manufacturers. They all claim, of course, to be the best. How then can a person make an informed hearing aid choice from all of this?

The key to selecting the most appropriate hearing aids is getting good professional help. Rather than spending your time investigating the different makes and models of hearing aids, you might be better served to acquaint yourself with the professionals in your area who sell them. Is their practice an established hearing aid center with a history of satisfied patients? Once you find a good professional, you can make use of their advice. The professionals will know which hearing aids work well and which ones are the most appropriate for a particular hearing loss and lifestyle.

A person might draw an analogy between selecting hearing aids for damaged ears and selecting the appropriate repair for a car that will not run. Most people know little or nothing about repairing cars and would not do well if left to find and repair the broken part themselves. The best option would be to find a good mechanic and let him or her solve the problem. To do this a person might ask his or her friends and family if there are any mechanics they know who do good work, how expensive they are, or how long they have been in business. Once a person finds a mechanic he or she has confidence in, however, the person lets the mechanic make the choices as to what needs repaired and how best to repair it. The car owner still has the choice to decline the repair, but the mechanic makes the technical decisions. Similarly, in selecting hearing aids a person's best option is to find a good professional and let him or her make the technical choices.

Don't hearing aids have poor sound quality?

The belief that hearing aids are not high-fidelity devices comes primarily from two sources. The first of these is from people who occasionally misunderstand with their hearing aids. They know they have a hearing loss, but feel that if they are not hearing perfectly with the hearing aids it must be the fault of the hearing aids. It is more often, however, a fault with the ears. Hearing aids can provide a very clear sound giving a person the best possible chance to hear, but the ears themselves may distort or incorrectly process what the person wants to hear. It is often in the act of trying hearing aids that a person discovers that his or her ears are distorting the sound. Without the hearing aids, not enough of any particular sound is heard for the person to be aware that it was not heard clearly. With hearing aids a person can hear words and other sounds well enough to be able to tell when there is distortion.

The second reason that hearing aids are reported to have poor sound quality is that they are adjusted to emphasize speech sounds. People wear hearing aids to be able to hear and better understand other people. Toward this end, some higher- or lower-pitched sounds may be reduced or blocked so that they will not interfere with speech understanding. The problem with this strategy is that the hearing aid frequency response that best compensates for a particular hearing loss may not always be the one that sounds the best. This becomes very apparent when listening to a symphony orchestra or rock concert with hearing aids. The music may not sound right. Some programmable and digital hearing aids have a special setting designed to faithfully reproduce music. Their primary setting, however, remains one that will emphasize speech.

Hearing aids usually have very good fidelity. They are set to compensate for a person's individual hearing loss and to help the person to hear what he or she most needs to hear. Unfortunately, even with perfect hearing aids there is no guarantee that a person's ears will correctly process everything or that the person will always be pleased with the balance of sounds that his or her hearing aids need to provide.

Maintenance

Tom Campbell brought his eighty-seven-year-old mother, Bertha, to our office for a hearing evaluation. Mrs. Campbell had been widowed many years before and lived by herself in her own home. She was no longer able to drive and depended on her son to take her to the grocery and to run other errands. Her hearing loss of more than ten years had become progressively worse. She wanted to hear family and friends and to hear the people she sees when her son takes her out. Mrs. Campbell thought it would be nice to be able to wear a hearing aid, but did not feel it would be practical for her. She understood that hearing aids use a battery, but believed that it could only be changed by a hearing aid professional. Getting out to have this routine maintenance would be too great a chore. She did not realize that she could easily change the battery herself and that replacement batteries were available at her grocery or could be ordered by mail through her hearing aid provider.

One simple misunderstanding about hearing aid maintenance left Mrs. Campbell to unnecessarily suffer her hearing loss for ten years. Although her particular misunderstanding was uncommon, there are other more frequent misunderstandings about hearing aid maintenance that prevent people from benefiting from hearing aids. These are examined here.

Wouldn't hearing aids be too complicated for me to work?
Hearing aids can range from being very simple to operate to very complex, depending on a user's wants and needs. An important part

of the hearing aid fitting process is to determine the level of complexity a person will be comfortable with and then to select hearing aids that will not exceed this level. If a person is comfortable adjusting the volume him or herself, he or she can have a volume control. If a person would like to be able to switch between different programs tailored for specific listening situations, he or she can have hearing aids with multiple memories. If a person would sometimes like to be able to focus on the people directly in front of him or her while at other times hear what is going on all around, the person could have hearing aids that can toggle between directional and multidirectional microphones. The list of possible hearing aid options is staggering, but need not be confusing. A person's audiologist or hearing instrument specialist can select the hearing aid options that will not only be understandable for a person to operate, but also appropriate for a person's specific hearing loss.

The elderly are the most likely to voice objections to hearing aids based on complexity. It is easy to understand how a person who has lived through all of the changes that have taken place over the last sixty, seventy, or eighty years might not be eager to learn about and have to cope with something else that is new. Understanding that many of the new hearing aids are like little computers, a person's initial reaction might be that hearing aids would likely be worse than the video cassette recorder he or she never learned to program or the television remote control with over one hundred buttons. Fortunately, advances in technology have made it easier rather than harder to use hearing aids.

Don't hearing aids need to be turned up and down all the time?

Hearing aids have traditionally been made with a volume control. This allows the wearer to turn things louder or softer, depending on his or her comfort level and hearing needs. Although these hearing aids can easily be adjusted, the average user does not need to turn them up and down all the time. Hearing aid wearers do, however, turn them up and down occasionally. They are likely to want more volume in a setting like a library where it is quiet and where people speak very softly. They are likely to want less volume in a setting like a bowling alley where it is very noisy and where people are speaking loud to get above the noise. They can set the volume to a level that is best for a particular situation. Once the volume is set, it can be left alone until they move on to a different situation where more or less volume would be wanted.

Going against the tradition of a user-adjustable volume control are hearing aids made with a preset volume. Years ago the only alternative to a user-adjustable volume control was no volume control. The hearing aid would be set to a fixed level. The volume chosen would tend to be a compromise between hearing well and not having things be too loud. This compromise resulted in hearing aids that were rarely at the optimal level for any specific situation. To prevent sounds from being too loud in any one setting, the hearing aids were frequently adjusted too low to be optimal. They were typically used for people who did not have the dexterity to operate a volume control or who could not use a volume control for some other reason. They were not the first choice of most audiologists and hearing instrument specialists.

As technology has progressed, hearing aids with a self-adjusting volume control are being chosen more frequently. Rather than the user listening with the hearing aids and deciding whether to adjust the volume, the hearing aids make this choice. The hearing aid analyzes the range of incoming sounds and determines the optimal volume moment by moment. This option is far superior to having a fixed volume and an excellent alternative to a manual volume control. This is an ideal solution for reducing the complexity of hearing aid use. The one drawback is that a hearing aid that adjusts the volume itself is usually more expensive than one that is adjusted manually.

Aren't there a lot of people who buy hearing aids but don't wear them?
The person voicing this concern is correct. There are people who buy hearing aids but don't wear them. They may feel the hearing aids do not help, that they do not help enough, or that they are uncomfortable or annoying. What many of these wearers may not recognize is that, like a finely tailored suit, hearing aids need tailoring by a professional. The settings programmed into new hearing aids are often only the starting point based on a person's particular hearing

loss. Individual listening demands and lifestyles almost always necessitate some fine-tuning. If the aids do not seem powerful enough, the gain can be increased. If they seem too loud, the overall gain can be turned down or the aid set to limit the maximum loudness. If the balance of pitches seems wrong or annoying, the frequency response can be adjusted. Similarly, it is not unusual even after taking an earmold impression for the fit to be off slightly, making an aid uncomfortable. If it is uncomfortable, this can be corrected. People who give up on their hearing aids without having these adjustments may be unnecessarily dissatisfied.

If hearing aids are tried and adjusted for the maximum possible benefit but are still found to be unsatisfactory, they should not be kept. A person should return to his or her hearing instrument specialist or audiologist and ask if there is a different kind of hearing aid that would work better. Hearing aid professionals sell their hearing aids with the understanding that they may be returned within a certain period of time if a person is dissatisfied. Hearing aid professionals understand that a person's experience with a set of hearing aids can sometimes be unsatisfactory, but still be productive in that his or her problems with the first ones can indicate a different type of hearing aid that might work better. If the new set of hearing aids is no better, they could also be returned.

Experienced hearing aid users can become dissatisfied if their hearing loss or listening demands change without compensatory adjustments being made to their hearing aids. There is a tendency to want to treat hearing aids as a one-time cure for hearing loss. Once a person has bought hearing aids, he or she feels that everything possible has been done and that there is no need for anything else. It is true that the person has taken the first and most important step to compensate for his or her hearing loss. Simply buying hearing aids, however, is not enough. It is also important for a hearing aid user to follow up by having the hearing aids periodically cleaned and by having subsequent hearing exams. Cleaning the hearing aids will prevent any buildup of wax that might block the sound coming from the hearing aids. The hearing tests ensure that any hearing change would be detected, making it possible for the hearing aids to be adjusted to compensate for this change.

The surest ways to become a person with unworn hearing aids is to keep hearing aids that cause dissatisfaction or not to seek adjustment for hearing aids that have become unsatisfactory.

How would I be able to tell the right aid from the left aid?

To maximize comfort, hearing aids are produced in slightly different shapes to fit each ear. It is necessary to know which is which. Fortunately, there is a simple trick to this that lets a person avoid the need for clairvoyance. The trick is to use color. Red is used to represent the right ear and blue to represent the left. There may either be a small colored dot next to the brand name on the aid or the entire portion of the hearing aid that is hidden in the canal may be colored. With one glance at the color on the aid, the problem of which ear to put it in is solved. Anyone who can figure out which shoe to put on which foot will usually succeed at figuring out which hearing aid to put in which ear.

Don't hearing aids get clogged with earwax and become disgusting?

Sometimes hearing aids do get clogged with wax, and when this happens, yes, they can be disgusting. The lining of the ear canal makes earwax. Some ears make a little wax and others make a whole lot. The earwax usually works its way out of the ear canal by itself and is not a problem. However, the physical process of putting a hearing aid into the ear can cause the hearing aid to scoop up some of this wax. It can either stick to the outer shell of the hearing aid or clog the opening where the sound is supposed to come out. If not cleaned occasionally, a hearing aid can get quite nasty.

Fortunately, it is not usually difficult to keep a hearing aid clean and free of earwax. The outer shell of the hearing aid can be wiped clean with a soft dry cloth. Since most hearing aids are very smooth and nonabsorbent, the earwax does not stick and comes off easily. If the wax gets into the opening where the sound comes out, it can also be removed. Most hearing aids come with a small wire loop that is designed to scoop out this wax. Audiologists and hearing instrument specialists should teach their patients how to do this so that hearing aid users can care for their own hearing aids. For most people these two steps of wiping off the hearing aids and scooping out any accumulated wax keep the hearing aids clean and working well.

In an ideal world the above two steps would take care of any earwax problems that might occur with hearing aids. Unfortunately, a few individuals produce so much earwax that the hearing aids tend to plug up faster than a person can clean them. For these people there are wax guards that can be built into the tip of the hearing aids. An alternate solution is disposable wax guards that stick to the end of the hearing aid and are then removed and replaced as they become dirty. If this is still not enough, an audiologist or hearing instrument specialist can professionally clean the hearing aids. There is no reason a person should have to live with hearing aids that are packed with wax and have become disgusting.

Don't hearing aids buzz and whistle all the time?

In certain instances hearing aids can make a buzzing or whistling sound that is heard by the wearer and others. This sound is called feedback. Feedback is produced by sound leaking around a hearing aid, finding its way back into the microphone, and being amplified again and again until all the hearing aid can do is scream at its maximum loudness.

There is always a little sound that manages to escape around the outside of a hearing aid, but this does not produce feedback as long as the sound does not go into the microphone. If a person covers up the hearing aid (for instance, with a hand, hat, or scarf), it is more likely to whistle because the escaping sound is reflected back into the hearing aid microphone to start the feedback cycle. A hearing aid may also whistle if turned very loud. This creates more sound pressure in the ear canal that may escape to reach the microphone. Although a hearing aid can be made to whistle in these ways, a properly functioning hearing aid should not whistle in normal use.

Three of the most common causes for hearing aids feeding back are a poor hearing aid fit, wax in the ear, or damage to the hearing aid shell or circuitry. If the fit of a hearing aid is off even a little bit, feedback is the usual result. A new hearing aid user with constant feedback can take his or her aid back to the fitter to have any subtle imperfections in the shape corrected. The feedback should cease once this is done. Persons with an older hearing aid can experience feedback if their ears have stretched a little bit over the years making the hearing aid fit loosely. These people can also return to their hearing aid fitter. In this case a thin coating can be put on the aid so that it will again fit snugly into the ear or a new, better-fitting shell can be made for the existing hearing aid components.

Excessive earwax is another cause of hearing aid feedback. If an ear becomes completely blocked with wax, the sound coming out of the hearing aid has nowhere to go except around the hearing aid and out of the ear. Even if there is only a little wax in the ear, it can still create a problem if the wax is directly in front of where the sound comes out of the hearing aid. The wax reflects the sound in the wrong direction, making it more likely to end up back in the hearing aid microphone. Having the wax removed by an ear specialist or using a prescription or nonprescription wax removal system on the ear will solve feedback problems due to earwax.

The above two causes for feedback—poor fit and excessive earwax—were caused by sound going around the hearing aid and into the microphone to be amplified again and again. A different form of feedback, termed *internal feedback,* results when the sound goes directly to the microphone through a damaged hearing aid case or when the feedback is due to an electronic fault. Dropping a hearing aid onto a hard surface such as a tile or concrete floor is the most common cause for the physical and electronic damage that produce internal feedback. Repairing a damaged aid will eliminate feedback caused by these internal problems.

Although feedback can be very annoying, it is unlikely to be harmful unless a person listens to it for long periods. Since it is annoying, this is doubtful to happen. Feedback is not the normal state for a hearing aid. If a hearing aid does produce feedback, it should be possible to fix it. Some of the newer hearing aids are smart enough to recognize when a feedback cycle is beginning and adjust themselves to prevent it from starting in the first place.

Could I use my hearing aids in Europe? The electricity is different there.

Anyone from the United States who has traveled to Europe will attest to the fact that it is not possible to simply go there and plug in the same electrical appliances. There can be a difference in both the voltage and in the type of current (alternating vs. direct). Without special adapters, a plug-in hair dryer, an electric razor, a computer, or any other electrical appliance might not work.

This difference in electrical systems between countries does not, however, affect the things that rely on a battery for their power. The battery makes them self-contained. A good example would be a battery-operated watch. It keeps supplying the same voltage it was designed to supply, and the watch keeps ticking away. Hearing aids are no different. Their batteries supply the needed power regardless of where a person takes them. The only time the difference in electricity might be a problem for someone with hearing aids would be if he or she has ones that use rechargeable batteries. In this case a special adapter might be needed for the charger to make it compatible with the local electricity.

Won't I be back where I am now after my hearing aids are old and worn out?

Given time, hearing aids do wear out and will eventually need to be replaced. Just like any other electronic device, hearing aids can break or eventually wear out. A rough estimate of the average life expectancy for a hearing aid might be five or six years. People who perspire a lot or work in a dirty or dusty environment may need to replace them sooner. Those who take good care of their hearing aids, do not perspire excessively, and are exposed to little moisture, dirt, or dust may have their hearing aids last much longer. In extreme cases a set of hearing aids might wear out in as little as two years or last more than a dozen years. Periodic cleaning and maintenance by a hearing aid professional can help to lengthen the useful life of a hearing aid and delay a person's returning to his or her starting point. The fact that hearing aids will eventually wear out, however, should not prevent a person from benefiting from hearing aids now.

Getting Used to Hearing Aids

Jason Bath was fifty-four years old when I first saw him as a patient. He had a previously documented sensorineural hearing loss caused by years of noise exposure while working as a self-employed carpenter. Although the hearing loss didn't cause him a problem at work, it did interfere with his family life and recreational activities. His fear was that he would spend a lot of money on hearing aids he might not get used to, and therefore, not use. This concern had kept him from seriously considering hearing aids during the three years since he was diagnosed with a hearing loss. Only after his brother became a successful hearing aid user did Mr. Bath reconsider his fear and seek help. Today, he is also a successful hearing aid user.

Mr. Bath's concern that he would not be able to adjust to hearing aids is common and accounts for many people continuing to suffer their hearing loss. This issue is discussed in the following pages.

I don't think I could ever get used to them.
There is often the fear that a person might buy but not use hearing aids because he or she could not get used to them. This concern merits attention because it does take a while to adjust to hearing aids. A person with hearing loss gets used to hearing the way he or she hears. No matter how hearing aids are adjusted, they will sound different from what a person is used to. Given time a person will become accustomed to hearing again if he or she wears the hearing aids. The person has to wear them, however, for this to happen.

Adjusting to something new or different is not a requirement reserved only for hearing aid use. Someone buying his or her first pair of eyeglasses may wonder how he or she will ever get used to everything being magnified or the appearance of standing ten feet tall. After a period of use, however, the glasses eventually seem natural.

Consider the process of getting used to a new car. At first it can be very frustrating. It is not like a person's old one. The headlight switch, climate controls, cruise control, seat adjustment, trunk release, and other features are not where the person expects them to be or do not work exactly the way the person is used to. After thousands of miles using this new car, however, it comes to seem as second nature to its owner. The owner gets used to its good and bad points: how it steers, how fast it accelerates, where its blind spots are, and so on. There is a definite learning curve that requires some adjustments on the driver's part. What makes the process of adjusting to a new car easier than adjusting to hearing aids are some differences in the assumptions people make for the two situations. People expect that it will take them a while to get used to and become comfortable with all of the idiosyncrasies of a new car. This degree of patience is less commonly seen in people adjusting to hearing with hearing aids. Additionally, few people doubt that they will ever get used to driving a new car.

Will my own voice sound unnatural with hearing aids?

It is common for people to report that their own voice sounds different with hearing aids. There are two major reasons for this. The first reason is that people are used to hearing themselves with a hearing loss. The hearing loss may be causing them to hear their own voice unusually soft or hear some of their own speech sounds better or worse than others. If you only hear low-pitched tones well, you may consider your voice to be deep and rich; if you hear high tones better, your voice will seem sharp and crisp. For the hearing-impaired person, this unnatural hearing is normal, and any change from this will appear strange or unfamiliar. The addition of hearing aids will make it possible for a person to hear a more even balance of sound that is necessary to understand speech. Even though the person hears and understands better, however, he or she may still complain that the sound is not natural. Fortunately, as a person wears the hearing aids and gets used to hearing this more even mix of speech sounds, it begins to sound more and more natural. Eventually a person comes to consider the more even mix of sounds heard with hearing aids to be natural. The absence of sound or uneven mix of sounds without hearing aids will then seem strange.

The second reason that a person's own voice may be perceived as unnatural with hearing aids has to do with why your own voice sounds different live versus recorded. When you speak, sound is conducted to your ear in two ways. The first is when sound waves leave your mouth and travel through the air to your ear. This is called air conduction. The second way sound reaches the ear is called bone conduction. This occurs when the vibrations of your voice are transmitted directly through the skull to the ear. The skull acts like the soundboard on a piano and shapes the sound slightly differently than the ear canal and middle ear. When listening to your voice on a tape recorder it is only the air-conducted sound that is heard. It sounds strange because it is not the combination of air- and bone-conducted sounds that you are used to. It is, however, the way others hear you!

Placing a hearing aid in the ear can also upset the usual balance of air- to bone-conducted sounds. In this case, the problem becomes too much bone-conducted sound and too little air-conducted sound as a person talks. Others will sound normal, but a person's own voice will seem to resonate in the ear. This phenomenon is known as the *occlusion effect* and can make it appear like you are talking in a barrel. You can easily simulate this effect by placing a finger in your ear canal while speaking aloud. There will be a noticeable change in the perception of your own voice. Fortunately, this effect can be minimized by changing the length of the hearing aid or by including an air vent in the design. Adjusting the frequency response of the aid can also help to compensate for this effect. The occlusion effect can be very distracting to a person when he or she first tries hearing aids. In time, however, a person can get used to this perceived change in the sound of his or her own voice even if nothing is done to minimize the effect.

Isn't there too much background noise with hearing aids?

The world is full of noise with or without hearing aids. Some of it a person might wish to hear and some of it he or she might not. A common expectation and misconception about hearing aids is that they will amplify only what a person wants to hear. Unfortunately, hearing aids don't work this way. Background noise is a subjective thing, and hearing aid designers cannot anticipate what, exactly, the wearer will want to hear at any given moment. What one person wants to hear could be background noise to another person. Hearing aids can be helpful, but they are not psychic.

Part of what makes background noise such a noticeable problem for a person trying hearing aids is that the person is probably no longer used to it. As someone's hearing gradually worsens over time, he or she becomes used to a quieter world. The person may not always hear what he or she would like, but there are fewer things that are distracting. Some compensatory measures further widen the gap between what a person would and would not like to hear. The television and radio are turned loud, as well as anything else that has a volume control. Family and friends learn to speak louder so they can be heard. Background noise does not interfere because the person does not hear it or hears very little of it. The person develops the impression that he or she is only hearing what should be heard: family, friends, and television or radio. The larger and more longstanding the hearing loss, the more entrenched this impression becomes.

People who try hearing aids often experience a rude shock: they suddenly hear everything. Sure they hear the person they are listening to, but that is not all they hear. They hear the furnace and the refrigerator running, faucets dripping, hinges squeaking, wind blowing, birds chirping, dogs barking, and much more. At first all of these sounds are distracting. They very much demand a person's attention because they are novel. With time, however, a person becomes used to living again in a world of sound. This initial reaction to noise is a hurdle that most new hearing aid users have to overcome. The more a person wears hearing aids and immerses himself or herself in sound, the quicker he or she will get over the hurdle.

People who had a hearing loss that was surgically restored often report this same experience. Right after surgery some of them emphatically state that they never would have had their operation if they had known that things would be so loud and that there would be so much noise. Once they get used to their new hearing level, however, these same people praise their good fortune. They are again part of the hearing world. They understand that it is always harder to hear in a background of noise, but they do not blame their surgeon for having made the world noisy.

Won't the wind be too loud with hearing aids?

This tends to be the golfer's complaint about hearing aids. People know from watching newscasters filing on-site hurricane reports that microphones can pick up unwanted wind noise. Newscasters will often cover the microphone with a large foam ball to protect it from the wind, but some of the wind noise may still come through. This same thing can happen with hearing aid microphones. The wind vibrates the microphone diaphragm and produces unwanted sound. Wind noise is most frequently a problem for hearing aid users who pursue relatively quiet outdoor activities. Besides golfing, wind noise can also be distracting for people who fish, hike, garden, or sit at outdoor sporting events.

The three solutions to hearing aid wind noise that may first come to mind are not the most practical. One of these would be to not wear hearing aids. This solution would solve the wind noise problem but would leave the hearing problem unsolved. The newscaster's solution of using a big foam ball over the microphone would eliminate most of the wind noise but might be considered aesthetically displeasing on a hearing aid. Another solution might be to wear a hat with earflaps or a scarf. This solution would effectively block the wind and reduce wind noise, but would also increase the risk of feedback. Luckily, many hearing aids can be built with a tiny windscreen that protects the microphone from the wind. It is unnoticeable or hardly noticeable (depending on the hearing aid design) and acts as the equivalent of the newscaster's foam ball. There are also some tricks of microphone placement that a manufacturer may employ to eliminate wind noise. For a potential hearing aid user, the key is to make sure that the audiologist or hearing instrument specialist takes into account whether wind noise would be a potential problem for the wearer's lifestyle or activities. If wind noise is likely to be a problem, the hearing aids can be designed to minimize it.

Infrequent Fears and Phobias

Caroline Trumbull was a fifty-seven-year-old divorcee who was seen at my office for a hearing evaluation. She came at the request of her children. It was obvious from her body language and the tone of her voice that she did not want to be in the office. Although she admitted suffering with a hearing loss for several years, she did not want to have anything done about it.

Mrs. Trumbull had an underlying fear of medical professionals. She told a story about being very dissatisfied with the fit of her dentures. Rightly or wrongly she blamed the dentist for poor work, for not caring, and for being only concerned about money. She had generalized the dissatisfaction with her dentures and dentist to all medical people and medical devices. She did not trust me and was not going to buy a hearing aid.

Given Mrs. Trumbull's experience with her dentist, it is perhaps not surprising that she approached an audiologist with skepticism. This wasn't a rational decision, but not all of us make entirely rational decisions about our health care. A number of fears and phobias exist regarding the use of hearing aids. Some of these can be paralyzing. They may prevent a person from trying hearing aids or from wearing ones he or she already has. The bases for these fears can be quite plausible. Other fears may appear unlikely or even silly. Plausible or not, each fear is a serious matter for the person involved. A number of these fears are presented and discussed here.

I am afraid of the examination.
Medical phobias are very common and often prevent people from seeking health care. Ear and hearing evaluations are not immune to this fact. A person may have had a bad experience with a physician or medical professional that he or she worries will be repeated. The person may have been prodded, poked, thumped, struck, injected, shocked, cut, siphoned, or something worse. Once too often he or she may have been told that something would not hurt even one little bit only to have it hurt quite a lot. If this kind of thing could happen with a family doctor, an eye doctor, or a dentist, why would someone be eager to risk having it happen in the ear?

Most people have never had a complete ear and hearing evaluation and do not know what to expect during one. It might be the most agonizing of all of the medical examinations possible. How would they know? They might just figure that it would be better not to find out.

Fortunately, having a hearing evaluation is not all that bad. Children approach the evaluation with the fear of getting a shot only to find out there is none. Adults may fear being hooked up to equipment that appears left over from the Spanish Inquisition. They instead find that the equipment is new and that their greatest risk of pain from the testing equipment is if they should trip over it or have it fall on them. If all medical evaluations and procedures were rated on a scale of one to ten with one being the easiest or gentlest and ten being the worst or most gruesome, having a hearing evaluation would rate a one or two. Anyone in need of this testing but fearful of having it should talk with his or her friends or relatives to find someone who has been through the process. They will confirm that it is not something to fear.

Aren't hearing aids unnatural?

Concerns about hearing aids being unnatural usually take two forms. The first is that a person should not be putting something unnatural into his or her body. The second is that hearing with hearing aids is an unnatural way to hear.

There is little point in arguing that hearing aids are natural. They are manufactured devices composed of plastics and electronics that do not occur in nature. While some people may see this as a problem, it should not be. The hearing aids are not being eaten, they are being worn. They may sit inside the ear canal, but they are still on the outside of the skin. They are not really "in" the body.

Other people feel it would be unnatural to hear with hearing aids. They listen to their own voice, other people talking, the sounds of nature, and other similar noises. These sounds come naturally into their ears without being reproduced or modified in any way. They feel that adding hearing aids would make the sounds appear artificial. What they overlook is how deeply technology is interwoven into everyday life. They already listen to people on the radio, television, and telephone. Listening to a person through hearing aids is not all that different from listening to sound reproduced through these other electronic devices. It is certainly no more un-natural or artificial.

Couldn't it give me brain cancer?

There has been a lot of concern over the past few years that the electromagnetic waves from power lines and the microwaves from cellular telephones may be giving people various cancers. The studies that have thus far been performed examining the health effects from these sources have not confirmed a risk. Nevertheless, not everyone has been reassured by these studies. Some people fear that this perceived danger might also apply to hearing aids.

Regardless of the validity of the perceived dangers of using wireless phones and of living in the vicinity of high-voltage power lines, I feel it can safely be said that these dangers do not apply to hearing aids. Hearing aids do not broadcast a signal like cellular phones. It is true that electricity is needed for hearing aids to work; however, the amount of electrical energy supplied by a hearing aid battery is so low that it poses no risk. Hearing aids have been in use for over fifty years, and there has never been a study implicating them as a cause for cancer. Furthermore, if there were a risk, it would have been most evident for early hearing aid wearers because their aids were less efficient and required more power.

Will a hearing aid interfere with my appliances?

Once in a while a person will buy an appliance or electronic device that interferes with another one of his or her appliances or electronic devices. An electronic children's game may interfere with television reception or call waiting on the telephone might complicate connecting to the Internet. Strong electromagnetic fields can seriously damage a pacemaker. As the world becomes populated with more and more electronic gadgets, the likelihood that one gadget will interfere with another becomes almost a certainty. Some people fear that by wearing hearing aids everywhere they go, it may cause problems with their television, radio, radar detector, computer, garage door opener, toaster, or other electronic device.

It is highly unlikely that hearing aids would affect other electronic devices. The hearing aids are not in physical contact with these devices; they do not broadcast strong radio signals; and their small batteries do not produce enough power to cause electrical interference. They certainly will not damage other devices.

Will a hearing aid set off metal detectors at the airport or alarms at a store checkout?

Although hearing aids are unlikely to set off alarms at an airport or other secure location, it can happen. The metal detectors in these places can sometimes detect the metal in the hearing aid circuitry or hearing aid battery. The detectors are much more likely to be set off, however, by the loose change in a person's pocket or by his or her car keys. People who are concerned that their hearing aid may set off one of these alarms can place their hearing aid in the little cup along with their change and car keys before passing through the metal detector. The guard will then return the personal items after they have passed through. Should a person forget and the metal detector go off, the worst that will happen is that the person will need to take out the aid and pass through the detector again: just the same as if it had been his or her car keys. Hearing aids will not set off alarms in department stores that are used to guard against theft.

Couldn't a wire come out of the hearing aid and puncture my eardrum?

Hearing aids contain many parts: wires, circuitry, batteries, microphones, and so on. Some potential hearing aid wearers worry that these parts might escape from the hearing aid and damage the ear. Although some of these parts—the wires or integrated circuits, for example—do contain sharp edges, they are normally well protected by the plastic shell of the hearing aid. This case acts as a barrier that prevents these parts from ever coming into contact with the skin of the ear canal. The portion of the hearing aid shell that touches the ear canal is molded as a single piece. It will not come apart from normal use. Unlike an old car that rusts and leaves pieces of itself behind, a hearing aid does not disintegrate.

Can hearing aids pick up radio and television stations?

Some people envision a scene not unlike that portrayed during an episode of the television show *Gilligan's Island* where two of the fillings in Gilligan's teeth were pushed together and began picking up radio stations. Day and night different radio stations came out of his mouth, depending on which way he turned his head. Some people fear the hearing aid equivalent of this.

While theoretically possible, it is highly unlikely that a hearing aid would pick up signals from radio and television stations. Hearing aids are not designed to receive radio waves. There is no antenna to pick up the signal and the circuitry is not designed to process it. To have any significant effect on a hearing aid the radio source would have to be very close or extremely powerful. Most hearing aid users are unlikely to encounter radio sources so strong or focused that they would interfere with their hearing aids.

Will I get electrocuted if the hearing aid gets wet?

Ideally, people should try to keep their hearing aids from getting wet. The reason is not that it is unsafe for the wearer, however, but that moisture is hard on hearing aids. The battery in a hearing aid contains such a small amount of power that the electricity it provides is harmless to an individual. Many people wear a similar battery everyday in their watch, but they do not fear electrocution when they discover the watch to be less waterproof than the warranty claimed. There is no more danger of electrocution from a hearing aid battery.

The real danger from water is the corrosion that it can produce within a hearing aid. This corrosion can damage or destroy the internal components. A person should not swim, shower, or walk in a pouring rain while wearing hearing aids. The hearing aids can be worn, however, while washing hands, doing the dishes, driving through a car wash, fishing, or pursuing other activities that do not get water directly on the hearing aids. A few drops of water from a light rain can usually be wiped off a hearing aid without any risk of damage. A hearing aid dropped into a sink full of water is a bigger problem. If something like this would occur, a person should immediately contact his or her hearing aid professional. The professional may provide instructions over the phone for drying out the aid. If the aid has been completely soaked with water, however, the professional will usually wish to see it as soon as possible to help dry it out.

Although water can cause permanent damage to a hearing aid, this risk can be minimized with quick care.

Couldn't a hearing aid battery leak acid into my ear?

This is an unfounded fear. Although the electrolyte traditionally used in automobile batteries is a liquid acid and has the potential to spill, the electrolyte used in hearing aid batteries is a solid or paste that will not leak. Furthermore, even if it were possible for a hearing aid battery to leak, the plastic shell of the hearing aid would protect the wearer. The battery poses no danger when used properly.

The one instance in which hearing aid batteries can be dangerous is if they are ingested. A person's digestive system can release the chemicals within a battery. Because of this, hearing aid batteries need to be kept out of the reach of children or pets that might eat them. I always tell people to keep batteries and medicines separate if they have a vision problem. If a hearing aid battery were to be ingested, the first action should be to call a poison control center or the number for the national battery hotline that is usually on the back of the battery pack.

Will the hearing aids cause me to hear voices?

Since the whole point of wearing hearing aids is to be able to hear voices better, the above statement might at first be puzzling. Why would a person not want to hear his or her own or other people's voices? This should be a good thing, right?

What is left unsaid in the above statement is that the voices these people are concerned about are not really there. They are concerned about what are called aural (hearing) hallucinations. While this concern is extremely uncommon in the general population, it is voiced occasionally by hearing-impaired persons with schizophrenia. They fear that hearing aids would make these internal voices loud and clear. Fortunately, while hearing aids may bring in other people's voices well, they should not cause a person with aural hallucinations to have clearer or more frequent hallucinations. If a person's irrational fear of this happening is so great that it might aggravate his or her overall condition, however, then this could be considered a valid reason for not wearing hearing aids.

Will dogs and cats attack me if the hearing aid whistles?

It has previously been explained that under some circumstances a hearing aid can produce feedback. This sound is not only noticeable to the wearer but also to those around him or her. If this whistling does occur, it tends to be loud and high-pitched. It can be quite annoying to people, but more so for dogs and cats because of their sensitive high-frequency hearing. Just as these animals will stop, pay attention, and sometimes be irritated by a dog whistle, they will often have a noticeable reaction to a whistling hearing aid. It is not uncommon for a dog or cat to chew a hearing aid that is left whistling on a counter. I have seen the results of this several times when patients had forgotten to turn their hearing aid off before setting it down. I have never seen a patient who was attacked by a dog or a cat, however, because his or her hearing aid was whistling.

Far-fetched objections.

There are potentially a limitless number of reasons for objecting to hearing aids. Some of them will appear very implausible, but still prevent a person from using hearing aids. One of these fears is that a hearing aid might freeze to the ear in winter. Although it is theoretically possible for a hearing aid to freeze to an ear, in real life it is highly unlikely. A person's body keeps the hearing aid warm so that there is no great temperature differential between the hearing aid and the ear canal. It may be very cold outside but the hearing aid remains warm.

Another implausible objection is that the CIA, the FBI, or someone else might use a hearing aid to monitor what a person does. Although designing an aid that could do this is not outside the realm of possibility, it is pretty far outside the range of probability.

One final example of a far-fetched fear would involve a phobia about technology. An extreme way this phobia has been manifested in regard to hearing aids is a person fearing a transformation into a cyborg. The very few individuals for whom this might be a concern can be reassured that hearing aids are something that are worn. They are not in any way integrated into the body.

Conclusion

Any one of the concerns expressed in this chapter could prevent a person from using hearing aids to compensate for his or her hearing loss. Usually there are multiple concerns that serve as obstacles. The most frequent worries are related to hearing aid performance. People question whether hearing aids work. There are other concerns about getting used to or taking care of hearing aids. People worry that dealing with hearing aids would be difficult or not worth the effort. Because most of these concerns are based on misinformation or a lack of information, they can usually be overcome with knowledge. Reassurance can be helpful when the concerns are due to fears or phobias. Most important for overcoming these concerns is not losing sight of the reasons a person would want to hear.

5 Benefits for a Hearing Aid User

With all of the doubts, hassles, and costs involved in getting hearing aids, it's worth repeating what's gained by wearing them. Every reason offered below eventually boils down to one simple issue: hearing aids allow you to hear. This includes hearing at home, at work, in the car, at the grocery, at the movies, and so on. The reason is to hear.

There is, however, a more subtle variation on this theme. The advanced course would stress that the reason is to hear better. This is an important distinction in that hearing aids do not restore perfect hearing. They help to compensate for a hearing loss. If a person's expectation of hearing aids is to help him or her to hear better, then hearing aids are likely to fulfill this expectation. If the expectation is to hear perfectly, however, then hearing aids may be a disappointment. This subtle difference in expectations helps to explain why people are sometimes dissatisfied with their hearing aids even when they are a great help.

Hearing loss limits a person in a variety of ways. Hearing aids can help to overcome these limitations. Hearing loss causes people to avoid activities or to participate less fully. Wearing hearing aids makes it possible for people to do more and to be more involved in the activities where they do participate.

Another way hearing loss affects a person is in his or her personal relationships. The inability to hear hampers the communication that serves as one of the foundations for these relations. Hearing aids improve a person's ability to interact with others. This interaction makes it easier to develop and to maintain relationships.

A person's ability to work can also be affected by hearing loss. It may prevent a person from being able to perform some jobs or make him or her unproductive in others. By improving communication, hearing aids help to make people more effective in many jobs. When a person has been barred from a job due to hearing loss, hearing aids can sometimes make it possible for the person to resume work.

Hearing aids can additionally improve safety on the job and in personal life. This includes more than being aware of fire alarms or carbon monoxide detectors. Being aware of what is going on around you or of things that do not sound the way they should often serves as the greatest clue to danger. Hearing aids can make this information available.

Finally, there are practical matters associated with hearing loss. Because the ability to hear is usually assumed, hearing loss can negatively impact many activities and interactions. This includes some things that are not really about hearing. Hearing aids can help a person to cope better when the expectation is hearing.

Described in this chapter are many instances where hearing aids can be used to improve a person's quality of life, personal relationships, job performance, safety, and ability to cope with practical matters.

Quality of Life

Expanding my universe.
People live in their own little universe. Making up this universe are the countless people and things with which they interact. There are the people they see, the ones they speak with on the phone, and the ones with whom they correspond. There are additionally the personalities they see on television or hear on the radio. Their universes are filled with gadgets that beep, buzz, sing, honk, pound, make other noises, and may even talk to them. Animals populate their universes. They bark, purr, moo, hiss, chirp, and make other sounds appropriate to their particular species. Raindrops falling, wind blowing, waves crashing, and leaves rustling are some of the sounds of nature that exist within their universes. These are but a few examples. The variety and depth of sounds is almost boundless. That is, if you can experience it.

Hearing loss limits your universe. You hear and understand fewer people. You are able to enjoy fewer television and radio programs. Microwave ovens may not beep and bees may not buzz. Cats may not purr and thunder may not rumble. The larger your hearing loss, the fewer people and things you can interact with. Your universe has shrunk.

One very good reason to wear hearing aids is to increase the size and quality of the universe that is available. By being able to hear more and hear easier, a person can do and experience more. A universe without the sound of ocean waves and birds singing is not as full. A universe in which a person cannot understand others can be a lonely one. Shouldn't a person have as grand a universe as possible?

Improving my self-confidence.

It may be hard to be confident when you are depending on hearing you cannot trust. A husband might proudly return from the store extolling the great bargain he got on a garden hose only to find that his wife had instead wanted Cheetos. A parent might find that he or she had at least temporarily traumatized his or her small daughter and all of her friends by giving an all-Bambi birthday party rather than the all-Barbie party the daughter had wanted. A movie lover might find that the classic movie he or she had special-ordered cost eighty dollars rather than the eighteen he or she had thought was quoted on the phone. It does not take too many instances such as these to wipe out the self-confidence of a person with hearing loss.

Wearing hearing aids can make it possible for you to hear better and to be more confident of what you hear. Once you are more confident of what you hear, it may be possible to be more confident in what you do.

Lowering my stress level.

Not hearing can be stressful. The above discussion noting how the problems caused by a hearing loss can affect self-confidence illustrates this. Every action a hearing-impaired person makes can go wrong. Will something misheard end up costing respect, money, a job, a marriage, a friendship, acceptance, or something else? It is all a gamble that could cost dearly. How you view yourself and how others view you may be on the line. Although there is sometimes concern that wearing hearing aids will be stressful, the reality is more often the reverse.

Avoiding being so tired at the end of the day.
Trying to hear and understand with impaired hearing is hard work. A person with hearing loss often has to expend a lot of effort concentrating on what is said. If a person puts forth this effort he or she may be able to hear well enough to get by, but be exhausted at the end of the day. Someone with normal hearing in the same situation would be able to hear what is said and what is going on around him or her without having to try. It wouldn't take concentration or particular effort. The person would simply hear.

Wearing hearing aids reduces the amount of effort a person has to put into hearing. A person may still concentrate on the things he or she really wants to hear, but the need to do this will not be as great. The end result of wearing hearing aids can be that a person is more relaxed and has more energy at the end of the day because he or she has not used it all trying to hear.

Laughing because a joke is funny.
Missing the punch line of a joke can be exasperating. Equally annoying can be missing part of the storyline so that the punch line makes no sense. This might occur around the water cooler at work or late at night watching the *Tonight Show* with a spouse. Not only does a person not hear and enjoy the joke, but he or she also has to decide how to respond to it. A person with hearing loss might not laugh because a joke is funny, but laugh because everyone else laughs. Rather than the joke being a moment for fun, it is a moment spent trying to respond appropriately and not embarrass oneself. This is hardly the intent of the joke teller.

Improving Personal Relationships

Improving my marriage.
Successful marriages are based on sharing and communication. Spoken language is one of the major tools that allow couples to do this. Communication is also essential for intimacy. Couples further discuss the weather, the kids, their day at work, stories in the newspaper, shows on television, plans for the weekend, and much more. They share not just their thoughts but also their feelings about all of these things.

The quickest way to discover how important sharing and communication are to a marriage is to look at marriages where communication has broken down. The end result is often unhappiness or divorce. Hearing loss may not be the leading cause for divorce, but the communication problems it causes can be a major contributing factor. A person with hearing loss becomes isolated from his or her spouse, and the spouse in turn feels isolated. Improving the hearing can stop the isolation, restore communication, and improve a marriage.

Being able to hear the vows at my son or daughter's wedding.
There are a number of personal events that can underscore the need for hearing aids. Not being able to hear the vows at a son or daughter's wedding (or your own for that matter!) might be one of these. After having spent years raising a child and sharing his or her joys and sorrows, it would be very difficult to feel left out of the wedding ceremony.

A wedding ceremony is difficult in that it is not a situation where a person can ask the participants to repeat. It might be possible to ask someone else what was said, but it would not be the same as having heard it first hand. Ideally, people would recognize this kind of upcoming event as a potential problem and take steps in advance to be able to hear. Unfortunately, it is often only after failing to hear in situations such as this that many people become motivated to do something about their hearing loss. This is good in that it gets an individual to do something about his or her hearing loss, but bad in that the person missed sharing in a one-time event that was very important.

Hearing my grandchildren.
Children can sometimes be difficult to hear and understand even for a person with normal hearing. They may be shy and speak quietly, say things incorrectly, substitute letters, and jump in a seemingly random manner from one idea to another. Hearing loss only adds to the difficulty. Since people with the most frequent pattern of hearing loss have the worst hearing at high pitches, children's high-pitched voices fall right into this area of weakest hearing.

Grandchildren present a dilemma in that although they can be very difficult to hear, there is usually a great desire on the part of grandparents to be able to hear them. Hearing grandchildren is much like hearing a son or daughter's wedding vows. It is something that should not be missed.

Participating during family gatherings.

Family gatherings are typically one of the first places that a person notices that he or she may have a hearing loss. A person is surrounded by the same family and friends he or she has known and conversed with for years. The person recognizes that although he or she used to be able to hear and understand friends and family in these surroundings, he or she now cannot.

Even if a person with hearing loss does not notice that he or she is having a problem, family members will. These are the people who have known the person for years. They know whether the person likes to talk about family, television, sports, or politics. If the person has always been involved and engaged, family and friends will notice if he or she withdraws and sits alone in a corner. If the person used to be able to hear and understand but now cannot, these changes will be noticed.

Participation is what is missed at these special times. You may miss being able to join in discussions and activities like you used to. Friends and family members will miss having you as an active part of their discussions and activities. Compensating for a hearing loss with hearing aids can make it easier to join in discussions and activities that would otherwise be missed. It helps you to participate again rather than sit on the sidelines.

Improving Job Performance

Performing a job more easily.

Most jobs require hearing. Insurance agents need to be able to hear their clients. Nurses need to be able to hear their patients. Teachers need to be able to hear their students. Construction workers need to be able to hear their foreman. People who work in fast-food restaurants need to be able to hear their customers and coworkers. Even artists who may not need hearing to create their art will usually need hearing to have a better chance to sell or promote their work.

Beyond the realization that a person needs to hear to perform many jobs is the realization that he or she needs to hear well to perform these jobs effectively. It is not enough that a fast-food worker hear that the customer wanted a hamburger. The person must also hear what the customer ordered on the burger and whether the customer wanted fries with that. It is not enough that a nurse hears what medication a physician has prescribed for a patient, but he or she must also correctly hear the dosage.

How much can a person afford to mishear and still perform his or her job well? How much harder does a person have to work to make up for the things he or she is not hearing? People who try hearing aids are often surprised to discover how much better and how much easier they can perform their jobs. The hearing aids take away much of the disadvantage their hearing loss had put them in at the workplace. Rather than trying to hear, their concern can instead be placed on trying to work.

Avoiding the need to ask "what" constantly and have people repeat.
Not hearing can leave a person with a choice. The person can pretend that he or she heard what was said or admit that it was not heard and needs to be repeated. If repeated, there is no guarantee that it will be understood the second time either. A person might ask someone else what was said, but this is equally frustrating and could again be misunderstood. Asking a friend or spouse to repeat what was said can become an aggravation for them. Worse is when this becomes a problem at work. A person cannot afford to become an aggravation to his or her customers, clients, or patients.

Wearing hearing aids is a more practical solution for understanding the first time, thus reducing the need for frequent requests for repetition.

Staying at the top of my game.
A person who has worked long and hard to reach the top of his or her profession usually has to continue to meet the expectations and challenges of others. Failure to do so can be personally and professionally

unfortunate. A company president, department director, lawyer, stockbroker, or technical expert cannot afford to appear weak, indecisive, or confused. Unfortunately, hearing loss can create these impressions and make it difficult for a person to remain at the top of his or her career. A board of directors may consider replacing a company president who does not appear involved. Employees may not be as productive or loyal to a manager whom they perceive as weak. If lawyers and stockbrokers appear befuddled, they will struggle to find and keep clients. By improving a person's ability to hear, hearing aids can help a person to stay at the top of his or her professional game.

Passing safety standards for a job.

Being able to hear is not only important in making it easier for a person to do his or her job, but in many cases, being able to hear is necessary to be able to perform a job safely. School bus drivers, for example, need to be able to hear the traffic, the sound of an oncoming train, the scream of a child who might have run in front of the bus, and much more. Other examples might include truck drivers and heavy equipment operators. For these professions and many others there are minimal hearing levels that are required before a person can obtain or renew a license to perform the job. Hearing levels worse than the minimum standard are unsafe and pose a risk to the worker or to others.

Fortunately, people are usually allowed to wear hearing aids to help them pass hearing-related safety standards. This is very similar to the people who have the restriction on their driver's license that they must wear eyeglasses or contact lenses. In each case, the focus is not on the amount of underlying disability, the focus is on meeting or exceeding a safety standard. Hearing aids make it possible for many people to obtain jobs or to continue in jobs that they could not safely perform without this help.

Other Safety Issues

Being able to hear house sounds.

The assumed goal in wearing hearing aids is usually to be able to understand speech. There are many everyday sounds, however, that are also important for you to hear. It is not even necessary for you to leave your home to find examples of this.

In and around the home there are problems that develop that are most easily detected early through hearing. A flexible water supply line for a sink or clothes washer may begin to drip, indicating an imminent failure. If a person can hear this, all that may be needed is to spend ten dollars for a new part. If a person cannot hear it, his or her first indication of a problem might be a room full of water. Similarly, the sound of a toilet running serves as an indicator for a needed adjustment or repair. Without this, a five-hundred-dollar water bill might be a person's first clue.

Aside from plumbing, there are other house sounds that might indicate potential problems. The sound of wind whistling through a closed door or window can indicate the need for caulking or insulation. A squealing sound from the furnace or air conditioner could indicate a blower motor in need of maintenance or replacement. A buzzing sound might indicate a swarm of bees that has taken up residence in a wall or under the house. Arcing sounds as a person turns on a light or appliance might indicate an electrical short circuit. A hissing sound could indicate a gas leak. Without hearing these early indicators a person might not know why the house was cold and drafty, why the furnace quit working, why there are bees everywhere, or why the house caught fire.

These are only a few of the things other than speech that a person might need to hear within a house. Even in a relatively quiet place such as a house, there can be a lot that should be heard.

Being able to hear traffic noise.
Although traffic noise is something that people would usually prefer not to hear, this does not mean that you would never want to hear it. Just as it is sometimes important to be able to hear different house sounds, it can be important to hear road noise. This is especially true for whoever is driving, but it can also be important for passengers who might warn their driver of an unseen hazard. Most people would hope that it is true for the drivers of the tractor-trailer rigs with whom they share the road.

Hearing loss might not prevent a person from hearing the blaring of a nearby car's horn, but it might cause him or her to miss other important sounds. A person might not hear the noise from the engine of a car cruising in the vehicle's blind spot. A person might react too slowly to a car stopping suddenly in front because the screeching of its tires was not heard. An approaching police car or fire engine might go unnoticed until it was too late to move safely out of the way. A person might drive too fast, turn too quickly, or try to stop in too short a distance for the weather conditions because the precipitation around him or her was mistaken for rain rather than sleet. Hearing the distinctive sound of ice hitting the car would have alerted the person that it was in fact sleet.

Being able to hear helps a person to be a safer and more secure driver. For anyone getting behind the wheel of a car or truck, what better reason could there be for wanting to hear?

Localizing sound.

Whenever the hearing is even a little bit different between a person's ears, it can be difficult to determine the direction of sounds. A person will hear a sound, but rather than being able to know immediately where it is coming from he or she will have to look for it. This can be amusing in some situations such as when a person may turn the whole way around in order to find the person who is speaking. It is much like when someone is standing beside a person and reaches behind the person to tap him or her on the opposite shoulder. The person turns the wrong way to search for the source of the tapping. Not knowing the direction of sound, however, can be a more serious problem and can be dangerous. It can be especially dangerous when a person has difficulty localizing sounds from traffic. One does not get too many second chances if he or she turns the wrong way to look for the sound from an approaching bus or truck.

Hearing aids can act to balance the volume of sounds between sides when there is a difference in the hearing ability between the ears. A person wearing traditional hearing aids can adjust the volume his or herself to obtain the best balance. Digital or programmable hearing aids can be adjusted by the hearing aid fitter to provide this balance. If the difference between ears is too great, it may not always be possible to obtain a perfect balance between ears, but the hearing aids can still be helpful for determining the direction of sounds.

Practical Matters

Understanding people who are soft-spoken.
Even a very mild hearing loss can make it difficult for a person to understand someone who is soft-spoken. Many consonant sounds for these persons are not loud enough to be heard. Some of the softest consonant sounds such as *h*, *th*, or *f* would be especially problematic. These tend to be very quiet sounds to begin with and may be even quieter for someone who is soft-spoken. A person with a mild hearing loss would know that a soft-spoken person is talking, but would have difficulty understanding the words because parts are missing. The listener could try to interpret what the speaker might have said by using the context of the sentence, but this can be a very hit-and-miss approach. It is not a substitute for hearing.

Wearing hearing aids can usually help a person with hearing loss to understand what is being said, even if it is fairly soft. Hearing aids boost these soft speech sounds and act to emphasize others that might be most affected by a particular hearing loss. The sound from hearing aids fills in the gaps in a person's hearing, allowing him or her to hear more of the speech rather than just pieces and parts. If a person can understand what is said when speech is loud, hearing aids can usually be used to help understand speech that is soft.

This is a practical matter because there can be soft-spoken people anywhere. Furthermore, it is often the listener's hearing loss that makes a person only appear to be soft-spoken.

Creating a better first impression.
Right or wrong, first impressions play a large part in how people view and relate to others. A person in a job interview may never recover from a bad first impression. The person's credentials may be impeccable but may fail to get him or her a job due to something done in the first thirty seconds of the interview that consciously or subconsciously turned off the interviewer. If a person creates a bad

impression on a first date, then a second date is unlikely. More often, a bad first impression will prevent a person getting a date in the first place. Similarly, casual acquaintances are unlikely to become close friends if a person creates a poor first impression. Why would they want to get to know a person better if they did not seem to like him or her in the first place?

Many things go into the making of a first impression. A few of these might include a person's looks, dress, height, posture, facial expression, or body language or whether the person maintains eye contact. If a person opens his or her mouth to speak, then vocabulary, accent, voice quality, knowledgeability, humor, and seeming intelligence are added to the mix. Imagine adding not hearing, misunderstanding, or responding inappropriately as part of the first impression. The greatest risk is not that an observer will think that there may be a hearing loss. The risk is that the lasting impression may be that the person does not pay attention, does not care, or is not too bright.

Not having to stare at everyone all the time.
Most people are able to lip-read at least a little bit, although they may not realize they are doing it. They may not always rely on lip reading, but will make use of this ability if a person is soft-spoken or if the television is turned too low for them to hear. They find lip reading helpful in difficult listening situations. Someone with hearing loss, however, is likely to use lip reading to help him or her understand even in easy listening situations. The greater the hearing loss, the more lip reading is used. If the person looks away, he or she may not understand what is said.

An unfortunate side effect of someone's extensively utilizing lip reading is that it may make the person being watched feel uncomfortable. He or she may have the feeling of being stared at. Although the process may appear to resemble maintaining eye contact, there is often a sense of concentration or intensity that is conveyed through expression or body language that goes beyond simple eye contact. Fortunately, wearing hearing aids can reduce a person's need to lipread and consequently the risk of making others feel uncomfortable.

Letting others know I have a hearing loss.

The current trend in hearing aids is to buy the smallest, least-visible hearing aids possible. Most people want to hide their hearing loss and anything that might be an indicator of it. If they cannot get hearing aids that are virtually invisible, they do not want them.

Bucking this trend of miniaturization and invisibility are a few rebels who wear hearing aids not just to hear well but so that others will know that they have a hearing problem. Rather than getting small or difficult-to-see hearing aids, they buy large behind-the-ear hearing aids that can easily be seen. They may even get them in bright colors or colors contrasting their hair to help them stand out. The reasoning is that if other people know that they have a hearing loss, these people may go a little bit out of their way to help them hear. People may speak a little bit louder, more slowly, or more distinctly. They may wait to talk until they are in the same room with the hearing-impaired person. They may make sure they are speaking directly to the person or be sure to get the person's attention before speaking. If something is misunderstood, they may be more willing to repeat. While the sight of hearing aids on someone else's ears may not motivate everyone to speak louder or more clearly, it motivates enough people that these larger or more colorful hearing aids can be especially helpful.

Visible hearing aids can also help people to avoid many of the unkind comments that are unfairly directed toward people with hearing loss. They are less likely to be told to "pay attention," to "quit daydreaming," or to "come back when they are willing to listen."

Saving my day.

There are some instances where the ability to answer a few simple questions can make the difference between having a good or a bad day. Imagine being in the process of passing through international customs and misunderstanding the questions of the customs officer. The official would have to decide whether English is really your native language. The agent would have to consider whether you are pausing to decide on the most plausible lie. Given enough time and patience, a customs official would sort this all out. Unfortunately, it will be your time and patience that the customs official is using.

Passing through customs is not the only scenario where using hearing aids might be a welcome alternative to the consequences of hearing loss. Rather than being questioned by a customs official, a person might instead be pulled over for suspicion of drunken driving and need to respond appropriately to a police officer. Worse consequences could result if a pharmacist misunderstands a prescription phoned in by a physician. Equally troubling would be an emergency telephone dispatcher who misheard where to send an ambulance. A scenario need not be as dramatic as these to still be troubling. Mishearing could also be a problem during a parent-teacher conference, travel planning, or financial decision making. It would not require too much thought for a person to come up with numerous other examples.

Being Able to Hear

A person could add one hundred more examples to this list of why a person might want hearing aids, but each one would only be another variation on the importance of hearing.

6 Benefits for Friends and Family

Hearing aids offer an obvious benefit to the wearer—the possibility of improved hearing. More often than not, however, friends or family members are the ones urging someone with hearing loss to buy hearing aids. Although they do so for many reasons, the reasons can usually be grouped into three general categories. The first category is related to their wishing to maintain or improve their relationship with the hearing-impaired person. They view hearing aids as a way to eliminate the burden imposed on the relationship by the hearing loss. The second category of reasons is related to convenience. Friends and family may recommend hearing aids because of the times the hearing loss inconveniences them. This is not, however, always the case. Friends and family recognize that it is usually the person with hearing loss who suffers the greatest inconvenience. Consequently, they may instead wish to eliminate the inconvenience for the hearing-impaired person. The last category of reasons is related to protection. Friends and family may want to protect the person from the negative consequences or stereotypes that can result from hearing loss. Regardless of the specific reason voiced for recommending hearing aids, in the end, family and friends all suggest hearing aids because they want to help.

Improving Relationships

The hearing loss affects them, too.
A common misconception is that only the person with a hearing loss is affected by not wearing hearing aids. This view is much like the idea of the victimless crime. A person may feel that no one else will be hurt if he or she does not wear hearing aids. In a physical sense this is usually true. There can be an exception such as a car accident

that might have been prevented if a warning sign had not gone unheard. Otherwise, a person's not hearing is unlikely to cause physical pain or suffering to others.

The risk of causing mental or psychological suffering is a different matter. The first source of this suffering is a real or imagined loss of control. Hearing loss can alter the entire dynamic of a relationship, family, group, or work situation. The person with hearing loss may not be able to do everything he or she once did. It may not be possible for him or her to do these things as effectively. Friends, family members, coworkers, or others may sense this weakness and feel that they have to take greater responsibility. This sets the stage for power struggles, role reversals, and so forth. It can cause stress, misunderstandings, and arguments. The frustration the hearing-impaired person experiences affects his or her mood and in turn the interactions with those around. Sometimes the hearing-impaired person is fully aware of this problem, which can increase the frustration over the loss of control.

The second source of mental suffering can be caused by the loss of shared activities. Hearing loss can limit what friends or family members can do or cause them to have to do more. A friend or spouse may no longer have a partner who is willing to accompany him or her to meetings, movies, or restaurants because the companion is afraid he or she will not hear. A friend or relative may instead find that these activities are no longer fun because he or she is now responsible for hearing all of the things their companion cannot.

A person could reasonably argue that victimless crime exists. Making the argument that choosing not to hear is victimless, however, is less reasonable. No matter how a person looks at this, someone else is almost always affected.

It hurts for them to watch.

It is difficult to watch a person suffer with hearing loss. It hurts to see a spouse unable to take part in conversations. It hurts to see a parent's embarrassment or frustration at misunderstanding important conversations. It hurts to see a friend not be able to participate in the things he or she used to enjoy. It hurts to see someone you care for withdraw and quit trying. Only an unfeeling person could not be affected by watching this.

Making private conversations possible.

Hearing loss makes it difficult to have private conversations in public places. Unless a person speaks up, he or she is unlikely to be heard by someone with hearing loss. The person with hearing loss will in turn speak loudly because he or she does not hear his or her own voice at its true volume. In either case, what is being said will be readily available to everyone.

If a person is aware that the hearing loss limits his or her ability to have private discussions, the person may avoid trying to have these discussions. If family or friends are aware of the problem, they may not try to initiate a private discussion. Imagine trying to have an intimate dinner at a fancy restaurant. How intimate can it be if you cannot discuss anything without everyone else in the restaurant hearing your conversation?

Perhaps more awkward than someone knowing that the ability to have private discussions is a problem is his or her not acknowledging that there is a problem. A person may try to share discreetly with a friend something very personal only to find that he or she has shared it with everyone present. It does not require too many episodes such as this to make someone with hearing loss recognize the problem here. Once this realization is made, a person often joins the first group who avoid trying to have private discussions in public.

Family and friends miss being able to have these private exchanges. It serves as a big motivation to suggest hearing aids.

Stopping a hearing-impaired person from monopolizing the conversation.

One way to deal with not being able to hear well is to prevent others from speaking or to control the topic of conversation so completely that there are very few possible replies to make. In the first case there is nothing that needs to be heard. In the second case there is such a limited number of likely possibilities for what was said that even a person with a significant hearing loss can usually make an appropriate response. From the viewpoint of a person with hearing loss, this can be a great coping strategy. The person always feels in control and seldom finds him or herself misunderstanding what was said. Not surprisingly, this coping strategy is used a lot, especially by people who are in denial about having a hearing loss. People use this strategy in their personal lives and also in their professional lives when they are in an occupation that will allow them to get away with it.

From the point of view of everyone but the person with hearing loss, this is a less-than-optimal way to deal with a hearing problem. These others are not going to want to be around a person who monopolizes every conversation. It becomes impossible to have a discussion with the person because all of the speech is in the form of a monologue. Friends and family would usually be much happier to have the person occasionally misunderstand what is said than never to be given the opportunity to talk. Even better would be to find a way to let the person hear so that there is no reason for him or her to use this annoying coping strategy.

Avoiding the accusation of mumbling.

Being accused of mumbling is a common reason for suggesting hearing aids. A woman with hearing loss may complain that her husband is mumbling. The husband may complain that he is talking as loud as possible. This creates some big arguments and many hard feelings. Each person feels that the other does not try and possibly does not care.

People who are trying their best to be heard do not appreciate being told that they are mumbling. Friends or family may suggest hearing aids to break this cycle of one party's blaming the other. Fortunately, wearing hearing aids lets a person with hearing loss take control of the situation. A wife can turn her hearing aids louder rather than having to depend on her husband's speaking louder.

Stopping a hearing-impaired person from appearing thoughtless.

It is important for a person to be aware of what is going on around him or her. This is true at work, around the house, in personal relationships, and for personal safety. In regard to family and friends, the concern is often being able to show common courtesy. This involves being aware of many simple things that may not seem so simple if overlooked. It involves not turning on the hot or cold water when a person should hear that his or her spouse is in the shower. It involves answering the doorbell because a person does not hear anyone else running to get it. It involves waiting to sign on to the Internet because a person can hear that his or her spouse is already on the phone. It involves a person being aware of these and other hearing-related things that would be of importance or concern to others.

Acting as though being out of sight also means being out of mind is not a good way for a person to demonstrate concern for others. Family or friends may suggest hearing aids as a way to help a person be more aware of what is going on around him or her and to help the person avoid appearing thoughtless.

Convenience

Eliminating the need to yell.
As a person's ability to hear gradually worsens, friends and family have a natural tendency to speak a little louder so that they can be heard and understood. At first, friends and family may not even be aware they are speaking louder. They just speak at the volume that is needed to carry on a conversation. As the hearing loss worsens, however, they reach a point that they can no longer speak comfortably at a level that is loud enough. Family and friends may be able to strain and speak at this volume for short periods of time, but it is uncomfortable. If they do this for long periods, they may suffer a sore throat or hoarseness afterward. Family and friends will feel like they have no choice but to yell.

Hearing aids can let the people around the wearer get back to a normal voice. Friends and family will no longer need to make up for the person's hearing loss. They won't have to yell.

To stop the person with hearing loss from yelling.
Friends and family aren't the only ones to speak up when a person can't hear. The person with hearing loss also speaks louder. The greater the hearing loss, the louder the person is likely to speak. Peo-

ple with severe hearing losses who do not wear hearing aids often yell everything they say because they cannot appropriately monitor their own voice. They will usually have the perception that they are talking at a normal volume. They will have no clue they are yelling. They commonly complain that their own voice is hoarse or raspy but fail to recognize that it is their own loud speech that is to blame.

Living with a yeller is not always a lot of fun. It is certainly not restful. Every day may start with a screamed "good morning" and every night end with an equally loud "good night." The middle of the day is no quieter. Standing close or far away, it does not necessarily matter.

Hearing aids can end the yelling and the problems it causes. Friends and family will not need to yell, and the hearing aid wearer will quit yelling once he or she hears the true volume of his or her voice.

Making it possible to turn down the television.
Television is an ideal device for a person with hearing loss. It can be turned up to whatever volume is needed, and a person can sit right in front so that lip reading can help. If the television is an expensive one, it may also have separate bass and treble controls that can be adjusted to compensate for a person's weakest areas of hearing. All that needs to be done is to adjust the television to the volume and tone that sounds best.

Turning the television this loud may not be a problem until the listener considers the other people living in the house. To them it can be a big problem. They may not mind watching *This Old House.* They might, however, mind the sound of each power tool appearing as if it were in the living room. Even the nightly news can be annoying if the television anchorperson sounds like he or she is screaming through a megaphone.

The use of hearing aids in this case is not just for the sake of the person with hearing loss. It is for the sanity of the people who live with or next to him or her. Once a television gets turned loud enough, a person had better believe that family and friends would recommend something to change this.

Making it possible to watch the television with the volume turned on.
A coping mechanism for watching television that some people with
a hearing loss use is to either turn the sound off or to watch only
programs where sound is not essential. The most common way people watch television without sound is to use closed captioning. This
lets them see the program and easily follow what is said. What they
may forget is that others would rather listen to the words than have
to read them.

The other way of watching television without sound is to watch
only those programs where the sound is not important or to insist
that it is more natural to watch some things without sound. Tele-
vised sporting events are the shows that people most often claim can
or should be watched without sound. They will argue that baseball,
golf, stock car racing, or other sports are meant to be watched without sound. Although these events may not always have a hearable
commentator if someone were to see them in person, they are not
without sound. Baseball has the crack of the bat and the roar of the
crowds. Golf has the sound of the swing and the ball falling in the
cup. Stock car racing has the roar of the engines and the screeching
of tires. Television captures these sounds and often adds background
and commentary to make them even more interesting. The sound is
an important and planned part of the program.

A person with hearing loss may believe that he or she can do
without the sound on many television programs. This person is unlikely, however, to be able to get others to give up the sound. These
others will want the volume turned on. This conflict can result in
added stress to a relationship that may already be strained due to the
hearing loss.

Reducing the need to repeat.
Friends and family of a person with hearing loss are often dismayed
to find that they have been reduced to the role of a parrot. Regardless of what is said, their function is to repeat it. They repeat what is
said on television. They repeat what is said at the movies. They repeat what the pastor says at church. They repeat what the waiter or
waitress says at a restaurant. They even have to repeat what they say.
Although it may be nice to be needed, it is no fun to be a slave to the

things that someone else cannot hear. It would be better if there were a way for the person to have heard it the first time. Seeing a way, friends or family will be quick to suggest it. They may even repeat it!

Reducing the need to face the hearing-impaired person to be heard.
People with hearing loss are more likely to hear and understand someone who is directly in front of them. This is true because the sound is going toward them and because the speaker's lip and body movements also convey meaning. When a person has hearing loss, friends and family quickly discover that they need to repeat less if they are facing the person. While this is great to reduce requested repetitions, it is bad in that people must stop what they are doing and go stand in front of the person to talk. This can be almost as aggravating as having to repeat. Given a choice, family and friends would generally prefer to have the person compensate for the hearing loss him or herself rather than having to change their own behavior.

To avoid being deafened by the radio after lending your car to a person with hearing loss.
This is much like the case of a person who turns up the volume on the television. The person adjusts the volume and tone to the level that sounds best to him or her, which is of course much too loud for someone with normal hearing. Making the situation with a car radio worse than that of a television is that the car radio is turned louder to get above the road noise. Furthermore, the sound is focused within the small space of the car. A rude awakening is in store for any normally hearing person who starts this car. It may sound like the front row during the loudest part of a rock concert or like a screaming match between radio personalities. Regardless of what is on the radio, the volume is unwanted. The car owner may rethink the liberal habit of lending his or her car to others, especially anyone with a hearing loss.

Reducing the aggravation caused by the person's hearing loss.
Friends and family of someone with hearing loss recognize the inconvenience. Some of this inconvenience may impact them, but

friends and family usually appreciate that it is the person with the hearing loss who suffers the brunt of the difficulty. Nevertheless, the inconvenience to friends and family can be considerable. When a hearing-impaired person refuses to acknowledge his or her hearing problem, this inconvenience for friends and family can instead become an aggravation. Right or wrong, family and friends are likely to view the person's refusal to face the hearing problem as the source of their inconvenience. Once this happens, relationships can be damaged or destroyed. The issue is not just the inconvenience of a hearing loss, it is where this inconvenience may lead.

Protection

Avoiding the need to support someone with hearing loss.
People with hearing loss do not always recognize all of the ways that the loss affects them. They may overlook how much it limits what they do or how much it limits what people may be willing to let them do. Family and friends see this and worry that even the person's ability to support himself or herself may be affected. They fear that if the person cannot hear well enough to do his or her job then their employer will have no reason to keep the person.

Fortunately, with the passage of the Americans with Disabilities Act it is rare that people get fired for developing hearing loss. This is of course when both the employer and the employee try to make reasonable accommodations to compensate for the disability. These accommodations may include the use of hearing aids or other assistive devices. Employers will often provide amplified telephones or headsets for phone secretaries, telemarketers, or transcribers. An employer may instead move a person to a different job that does not require good hearing. If hearing aids are needed, however, they are usually considered a personal device that the employee would have to buy.

A person might ask whether it is possible to be fired for not wearing hearing aids. The answer to this in theory is no. The answer in the real world is yes. A certain level of hearing is required to safely and legally perform some jobs. If a school bus driver cannot meet the minimum hearing standard for driving the bus without hearing aids, then he or she will not be permitted to drive without hearing aids. Trying to do so would result in being fired.

Being fired for not wearing hearing aids, however, usually takes a less direct route. A real-estate saleswoman who mishears the wants and needs of her clients will likely be fired due to poor sales performance. A cook who continually makes the wrong foods may be fired for inattention. A purchasing agent who signs deals based on misheard price quotes may be fired for incompetence. People such as these are not fired for having a hearing loss, but for the consequences of the loss. The employers of these individuals would not fire them for failing to wear hearing aids. They would be unlikely to be aware their employees had a hearing loss. This would be especially true for the many employees who deny any hearing problem. With very few exceptions, people cannot legally be fired from a job because of a hearing loss. They are, however, frequently fired as an indirect result of their hearing loss.

Hearing is so important in the workplace that private, state, and federal agencies will sometimes pay for an evaluation to determine whether hearing aids could help to make a person employable. If the evaluation shows the need for hearing aids, the agencies may even pay for them. The determination of need is usually based on the severity of the hearing loss and on financial need. Providing these tools so that people can earn a living makes a lot of sense in the long run. It is better to help a person to be a productive taxpayer than to have them unemployed and collecting disability or welfare. Family and friends of a person with hearing loss would rather see the person take whatever steps are needed to become or remain gainfully employed than possibly falling through the cracks in the welfare system and possibly becoming their own responsibility.

Reducing the appearance and reality of handicap.
As was discussed previously, many people do not want to wear hearing aids because they fear they will appear to have a handicap. Nothing makes a person look more handicapped, however, than being handicapped. The appearance of hearing aids is insignificant compared to not hearing.

Family and friends of a person with hearing loss are aware of the handicap. They know the person struggles to hear and to participate. They see them withdraw and not participate. They also view hearing aids as a way to prevent hearing loss from incapacitating their loved one. Of course they are going to suggest them.

Saving them from themselves.

Just as a simple potion could transform Dr. Jekyll into Mr. Hyde, there are things that can turn a normally happy and easygoing person into a monster. This transformation is frequently seen with someone who is trying to quit smoking. Being sick, tired, overworked, or stressed have all been seen to lead to this transformation. So too has hearing loss. Living with the limitations and stress that a hearing loss imposes turns many people nasty. Friends and relatives get tired of dealing with this and want the return of the kind, considerate person they know and love. They suggest hearing aids in the hope that this will save them from the monster.

A Final Word on the Suggestion of Trying Hearing Aids

The suggestion to try hearing aids by family or friends is rarely greeted with enthusiasm. This is true regardless of whether hearing aids are recommended to strengthen a relationship, for convenience, or as a form of protection. There can be a certain us-against-them mentality that develops between a person with hearing loss who does not want to buy hearing aids and between friends, relatives, or coworkers who think that hearing aids would help. This struggle can involve any of the issues of denial, anger, bargaining, privacy, power, autonomy, and so forth that have already been discussed. The whole issue of hearing is sometimes lost to the greater concern of who will win and who will lose. This point is illustrated by the words of a woman with hearing loss who said about her family's wanting her to have hearing aids, "I won't give them the satisfaction." The argument had moved beyond hearing. She wanted to win!

The very nature of how a hearing loss affects a person and their relationships with friends and family makes it impossible for one party to win while the other loses. Either they both win or both lose. If a person resists using hearing aids then all suffer. If a person uses hearing aids and does well, then all win.

It is highly unlikely that family or friends would suggest hearing aids only so that they could later say, "I told you so." If this were the sole purpose, family or friends would pick something quicker, easier, or cheaper that they could use to win this game. If family or friends are pushing hearing aids, it is not to say, "I told you so." It is because they want to help.

7 Hearing Aids 101

Information is essential for a person to be able to decide between the different hearing aids and hearing aid options that are available. Are smaller hearing aids better than larger hearing aids? Is newer better? Is more expensive better? What makes a digital hearing aid different from a regular aid? The information necessary to answer these and other questions that would be helpful to a potential hearing aid user are discussed in this chapter. Basic information about hearing aid styles and circuitry is provided first. Potentially useful options and add-ons are discussed next. Finally, information is provided to help a person decide among these options.

About Hearing Aids

Hearing Aid Styles

The term *style* in regards to hearing aids is a reference to its physical size, how it looks, or where it is worn in or on the ear. The style of hearing aid a person can wear is influenced by the severity of the hearing loss, the shape of the ear canal, a person's dexterity, and what he or she finds cosmetically acceptable. Generally speaking, the larger the hearing loss, the larger the hearing aid will need to be. The increased size allows more room for circuitry and a larger battery to power it. It also allows for more surface contact between the ear and the hearing aid, making it harder for the amplified sound to leak out of the ear and be lost. Larger hearing aids are also better for people with poor dexterity. Those more concerned with cosmetics might choose smaller hearing aids. Although there can be advantages for one style over another, there is not usually a difference in quality among styles.

The most common in-the-ear hearing aid styles along with placement of the landmarks on each hearing aid are shown in figure 7.1. A behind-the-ear hearing aid is shown in figure 7.2. The different hearing aid sizes ranging from smallest to largest are described below.

Completely-in-the-Canal (CIC) Hearing Aid. This is the smallest of the canal hearing aids and the one that is most frequently advertised by hearing aid manufacturers. It fits far enough into the ear canal that it is very difficult for other people to see. One distinguishing feature of this style of aid is that it has a small removal cord attached that looks like monofilament fishing line. This cord allows the aid to be easily removed from the ear.

Mini Canal Hearing Aid. This aid is slightly larger than a CIC hearing aid and does not sit quite as deeply in the ear canal. The slightly larger size often permits the aid to have a volume or other

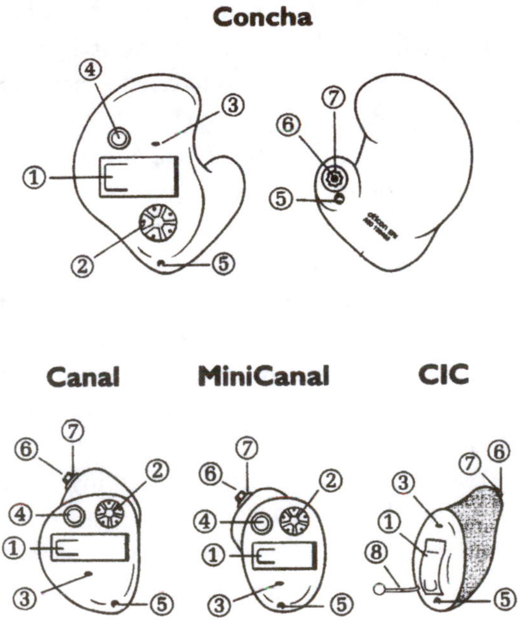

Figure 7.1 Sizes and landmarks of ITE hearing aids. Landmarks: 1—Battery door, 2—Volume control, 3—Microphone opening, 4—Telecoil switch, 5—Air vent, 6—Sound outlet, 7—Wax guard, 8—Removal string. Courtesy of Oticon.

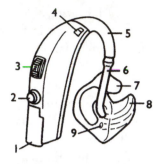

Figure 7.2. Landmarks of a BTE hearing aid with earmold. Landmarks:
1—Battery door, 2—Telecoil switch, 3—Volume control, 4—Microphone
opening, 5—Ear hook, 6—Plastic tubing, 7—Earmold, 8—Sound outlet,
9—Air vent. Courtesy of Oticon.

user-adjustable control. A volume control is not usually practical on a CIC aid due to its small size and placement in the ear.

Canal Hearing Aid. This hearing aid fits entirely in the ear canal. It is a little larger than the CIC and mini canal hearing aid. The outermost edge sits about flush with the opening to the ear canal. While larger than the CIC and mini canal, it is still not very noticeable. The little bump in front of the ear canal (the tragus) tends to hide the hearing aid from someone facing the hearing aid wearer. From the back the aid is hidden by the outer part of the ear. The aid is usually visible only to someone standing beside the person who is looking directly into the ear. If this were to happen, however, the natural tendency of the person wearing the aid would be to turn to face the other person. The aid would then be hidden by the tragus.

Half-Shell Hearing Aid (not shown). This hearing aid is only slightly larger than a canal aid. In addition to filling the ear canal, the aid also extends out a little way into the lower part of the outer ear. If the ear canal is an unusual size or shape, this extension can help to hold the hearing aid in place. It may also increase the amount of surface contact between the aid and the ear, which is important for keeping sound in the ear.

In-the-Ear (ITE) Hearing Aid. This is a general term used to refer to any hearing aid that fits entirely into the ear. It is also used to refer to the largest of the in-the-ear hearing aids that completely fill up the bowl-shaped portion of a person's ear. This style of hearing aid is generally used for more severe hearing losses than can easily be corrected with smaller hearing aids. The larger size permits greater room for circuitry and a larger battery. The increased surface contact between the aid and the ear make it even harder for the amplified sound to escape the ear. An ITE aid is also referred to as a full-shell or concha aid.

Behind-the-Ear (BTE) Hearing Aid. The battery and electronics in this form of hearing aid hang behind the ear. Sound is carried from the body of the aid through a small tube to an earmold that fits in the ear. This hearing aid is the best choice for people with severe hearing losses. Like the ITE, it has room for more circuitry and a larger battery. The ample surface contact between the earmold and the ear keeps sound from escaping at least as well as and sometimes better than an ITE aid. Also, by placing the microphone on the body of the aid at the top of the ear, it is less likely for any sound that does escape to find its way into the microphone and cause the aid to whistle. This is also the hearing aid of choice for use with children. The advantage is that, as they grow, all that needs to be replaced is the earmold. Parents don't have to keep buying new hearing aids or have them remade as would need to be done with any of the in-the-ear styles. Some people consider this style of aid to be old-fashioned or unsophisticated. While it is true that this may be an older style of hearing aid, they are as technologically advanced as the smaller hearing aids.

Eyeglass Hearing Aid (not shown). This is a style of hearing aid in which the working parts are built into a person's eyeglass frames. The sound is carried through a small clear tube to an earmold worn in one or both ears. It is essentially a BTE hearing aid that is built into a person's glasses. Although once fairly popular, this style has fallen out of favor. The most obvious reason for this is their cosmetic disadvantage when compared with the ITE and many of the smaller BTE hearing aids. Furthermore, the large plastic eyeglass frames that can best house these aids are not currently in fashion.

Body Aid (not shown). This is the largest and most powerful of hearing aids. The electronics for the hearing aid and the battery that powers it are housed in a small case about the size of a cigarette pack that is worn somewhere on the body. The sound is carried through a small wire to an earpiece. This style of hearing aid is uncommon today because advances in technology have made it possible to compensate for most hearing losses by using one of the smaller hearing aids already discussed. This style of hearing aid is still available, however, and may be the best option for people with extremely severe or profound hearing loss.

Implantable Hearing Aids

Some people would prefer to have a hearing aid that is not just worn but implanted in the body. They envision it to be permanent, carefree, and invisible. What is wanted is a technological fix that pushes the limits of available technology. The major obstacle to a completely implantable aid is how to supply it with power. Some kind of battery is needed. It would not be very practical to use a conventional hearing aid battery because this would necessitate cutting a person open every couple of weeks to change it. A longer-life battery might be used but it would still need to be replaced periodically. Rechargeable batteries might be an option, but then some method of charging them while still within the body must be employed. Still, even rechargeable batteries wear out eventually.

Although not entirely implantable, there are hearing devices currently available that have implantable parts. The implanted portion tends to be a small magnet or vibrator that is attached to one of the ossicles in the middle ear. Each of these acts to move the ear bones back and forth in response to sound allowing a person to hear. The middle ear magnet is moved through magnetic induction (the force of one magnet moving another) by a portion of the hearing aid worn externally behind the ear or in the ear canal. The middle ear vibrator moves the ossicles in much the same way as the coil in a speaker moves its cone. In each of these cases the battery that powers the aid is housed in the externally worn part so that it may be changed easily. The sound produced by one of these semi-implantable hearing aids has been reported to be as good if not better than a conventional hearing aid. Surgery is involved, however, and the price can be prohibitive. This technology does help a person to hear, but it is not the permanent, carefree, and invisible solution that is wishfully envisioned.

Circuitry Options

There is more to selecting a hearing aid than deciding how big it should be. An equally important if not greater concern is what is inside. Two hearing aids made by the same manufacturer that look absolutely identical can perform very differently depending on the circuitry. Similarly, two dissimilar styles or brands of hearing aids may perform alike if they have similar circuitry. The type of circuitry dictates the ways in which a hearing aid can perform and has more impact on price than either the style or the brand name.

A list of the hearing aid circuitry options claimed by all of the different hearing aid manufacturers would be rather lengthy. Most of the hearing aid manufacturers would list at least several different circuits or circuitry options for which they claim proprietary rights. The number of choices might seem overwhelming to the average person. Fortunately, it is possible to narrow the number of hearing aid circuits down to a few general types. These are listed below.

Analog Hearing Aid. This is sometimes called a conventional, standard, or traditional hearing aid. Similar to other hearing aids it has a microphone, an amplifier, and a receiver that deliver sound to the ear. All of the sound in an analog hearing aid is processed as a voltage just as is done in a radio or in older stereo equipment. A method called selective amplification is used to determine how much any frequency is amplified. The greater the hearing loss at any particular frequency, the more amplification will be needed at that frequency. This combination of analog technology and selective amplification can provide a very clear and accurate reproduction of sound. The problem is keeping sounds within an audible, natural seeming, and comfortable range. If a person turns the aid up loud enough to hear soft sounds, then loud sounds may be too loud. If the aid is turned down so that loud sounds will not be overly loud, then soft sounds may not be heard. While it is possible to keep sounds from becoming too loud by having a loudness cutoff point or limiting the loudness growth rate, there are limits to this technology which may still leave sounds uncomfortably loud or unnatural sounding.

Digital Hearing Aid. This kind of hearing aid processes sound as numbers. It acts much like a mini computer. Digital hearing aids are programmed using more complex methods of selective amplification than are possible with analog hearing aids. This allows the aids to monitor incoming sounds to keep them in an audible and comfortable range. The hearing aids can be made to modify sound in almost an infinite number of ways simply by changing numbers within their program. This ability to modify sounds gives digital aids an advantage over analog hearing aids. Digital hearing aids can also be subtly adjusted to account for individual preferences in how things sound. The ultimate in digital hearing aids (an open-platform hearing aid) can be set not only for different hearing losses but also has the future potential to be reprogrammed to code or filter speech in ways that may not even have been thought of yet.

Programmable Hearing Aid. Although digital hearing aids are sometimes referred to as being programmable, the term *programmable hearing aid* is generally used to denote a hybrid that has parts of both an analog aid and a digital one. It has digital components that allow it to be programmed on a computer, but the underlying amplifier is analog. This combination of technology allows for more flexibility in adjusting to individual hearing losses and listening preferences than may be possible with an analog aid but not as much flexibility as can be obtained by a fully digital aid. People who want more than can be provided by conventional hearing aids but who cannot afford digital aids often choose programmable aids as a compromise.

Channels and Bands

Differentiating hearing aids within a particular circuit type are the number of channels or bands it has. A two-channel hearing aid would divide incoming sounds into low and high frequencies. A four-channel hearing aid might divide incoming sounds into low, medium, high, and very high frequencies. It is possible to adjust how sounds are amplified within each channel, and this adjustment is independent of the other channels. Bands are subdivisions within a channel. Individual bands can also be adjusted, but they are not always completely independent of each other. This means that turning up or down the gain in one band may also affect the one next to it.

The more channels and bands a hearing aid has, the more adjustable it is.

Conventional analog hearing aids are customarily single-channel devices that can be modestly adjusted at low- or high-frequency bands. Programmable hearing aids typically have one or two channels. The most basic single-channel programmable aids are usually at least as adjustable as the best conventional aids. Two-channel programmable hearing aids are more adjustable. Digital hearing aids usually have at least two channels, and a few have ten or more. These channels are often subdivided into several bands that allow for very fine adjustments.

More channels or bands denote a more sophisticated hearing aid. It also implies greater flexibility to compensate for an individual's hearing loss.

Specialized Hearing Aids

In addition to the previously described styles of hearing aids, there are hearing aids designed for very specific kinds of hearing loss. These hearing aids would not be appropriate for the average person with hearing loss. They can, however, provide help to people with less-common hearing losses.

Contralateral Routing of Signal (CROS) Hearing Aid. This aid is designed for a person with normal hearing in one ear and a total hearing loss in the other. Part of the hearing aid is worn on the non-hearing ear and transmits sound to a part worn on the normal-hearing ear. By transmitting sound to the opposite ear, the hearing aid effectively keeps a person's head from getting in the way of sound trying to reach their good ear. A CROS hearing aid can help a person to hear better, but it does not restore hearing to the "dead" ear.

This is an important alternative to traditional hearing aids. If there is no awareness of sound or word understanding in the bad ear, then making sounds louder with a regular-hearing aid will not make any difference. The person must depend solely on his or her better-hearing ear. This may work fairly well when sounds are coming from the front or from the better-hearing side. When sounds are coming from the opposite side, however, a person's head gets in the way of the good ear. This "head shadow" effect makes it difficult to hear some of the softer consonant sounds when they are directed toward a person's bad side, even in an otherwise ideal listening situation. A CROS aid overcomes this.

Bilateral Contralateral Routing of Signal (BICROS) Hearing Aid. This is a special version of a CROS hearing aid that is designed for a person with a partial hearing loss in one ear and a total hearing loss in the other. Part of the hearing aid is worn on the non-hearing ear and transmits the sound across to the corresponding part on the better-hearing ear. The part on the better-hearing ear amplifies sound from this side and from the non-hearing side. All this sound is combined and sent into the better-hearing ear. It is a regular hearing aid and a CROS hearing aid all rolled into one.

Bone Conduction Hearing Aid. This kind of hearing aid can be an option for persons with normal-hearing nerves who have a problem with their outer or middle ear. Their problem might be the congenital absence or malformation of an outer ear or of the middle ear bones. Their problem might instead be acquired later, such as a perforated eardrum or ear bones damaged from trauma, infection, or disease. A bone conduction hearing aid bypasses these problems. It works by gently vibrating the skull, which transmits the sound through the bones of the skull to the hearing nerves. It can allow a person with normal-hearing nerves to hear regardless of the amount of peripheral damage or malformation.

Custom versus Non-Custom Hearing Aids

The majority of hearing aids in use are custom made specifically for their user. Impressions are taken of their wearer's ears, and the hearing aids are made to fit this exact shape. Similarly, the electronics and the way these electronics are adjusted are specific to the individual user. While all of this special care makes for hearing aids that are individually optimized for a person's ears and hearing loss, it also makes for a high price tag.

Eliminating all of this customization is one strategy to reduce the cost. Rather than each hearing aid having to be made and adjusted individually, many identical units are produced. Since a high-frequency hearing loss is the most common, the electronics are usually designed to compensate for a hearing loss in this frequency range. The shape of the aid is normally designed to fit within an adult ear canal and may be made of a soft material or have an adapter to make up for irregularities in the fit. A few are made to fit behind the ear similar to a BTE aid. There may also be a volume control to allow the user to set the hearing aid to the level he or she finds most comfortable. While these one-size-fits-all hearing aids can be helpful to many people at a greatly reduced cost, their fit and performance may not be optimal. One-size-fits-all designs work well for things such as nightshirts. But we would not think of buying a suit or evening gown this way. While a one-size-fits-all suit or evening gown would keep us decent, few would argue that it would be as good as one that is tailored to fit. The argument is similar for non-custom hearing aids. In fact, many of these cannot legally be sold as "hearing aids." Some other term must be used. Still, they are considered here as a form of hearing aid because this is the public perception.

Although non-custom hearing aids may not be the optimal choice for an individual, they are still an option. A person may have a hearing loss and an ear canal shape that matches up well with the design and shape of these devices. If not, a person may instead be willing to trade a little bit of comfort or performance for the much smaller price. Anyone wanting to try these non-custom hearing aids can usually find them advertised for mail order in newspapers and magazines. The option of a money-back guarantee is customary if a person is dissatisfied for any reason.

Disposable Hearing Aids

Disposable hearing aids have some of the same attributes as non-custom hearing aids. The approach can also be thought of as one-size-fits-all or at most a-few-sizes-fit-all. As with other non-custom hearing aids the goal is to produce so many copies of the same hearing aid that the price is dramatically lowered. In this case the goal is to drive the price so low that a hearing aid can be used for a short while and thrown away. It worked for disposable contact lenses. Why not hearing aids? Although the long-term cost of buying disposable hearing aid after disposable hearing aid eventually adds up, it does not require the large initial outlay that it takes to buy a custom-made hearing aid. This makes the prospect of purchasing a disposable aid less frightening. A person may figure that if it does not work to their satisfaction, he or she will simply not buy any more.

Disposable hearing aids can be used as a permanent solution to a person's hearing loss as long as he or she does not mind buying multiple hearing aids. At the time of this writing, disposable hearing aids can be purchased only from audiologists and hearing instrument specialists. A person goes to a hearing professional for an initial hearing evaluation and to select a pair of disposable hearing aids that are appropriate for him or her. Replacement hearing aids can be purchased without a repeat evaluation; however, yearly evaluations are recommended to ensure that the hearing aids being purchased remain appropriate.

The long-term cost of disposable versus custom hearing aids is arguable. If a person assumes that the custom aids will last many years and have few repairs, then they may cost less in the long run. If, however, a person assumes a shorter lifespan with multiple repairs and includes things like the cost of batteries and possibly hearing aid insurance, then disposables may cost less.

Disposable hearing aids can also be used as a short-term solution to a hearing problem. A person with a correctable ear problem might use a disposable aid until surgery can be scheduled to correct the hearing problem. A person might buy a disposable aid to replace a broken hearing aid temporarily while it is being repaired. A disposable hearing aid might be kept on hand as a spare just in case a problem might develop with a regular hearing aid. A disposable hearing aid is also a good alternative for times when a person is engaging in activities that might damage their more expensive custom hearing aid. The risk of hearing aid damage from white water rafting might be a good example.

Personal Amplifiers

In terms of both cosmetics and technological sophistication this option might be considered a last choice. For a few people, however, it is an effective, low-cost solution to a hearing problem. This device looks very much like a small portable radio. It has a small box that is carried or worn somewhere on the body and a set of earphones that go over the ears. Rather than receiving radio stations, the unit picks up and amplifies sound. It has a volume control and sometimes a balance control so it can be adjusted separately for each ear. A few even have a small graphic equalizer so that a person can select the pitches he or she wants emphasized. A personal amplifier can be ordered from an audiologist or hearing instrument specialist but can usually be obtained less expensively from a retail electronics store.

A personal amplifier can be a good choice for someone who cannot afford hearing aids. A personal amplifier can also be a good choice for someone who only wants help occasionally but does not feel this occasional use warrants the cost of hearing aids. An example of this might be a retired person who lives alone and only wants help when his or her children or grandchildren visit. The large size of the device additionally makes this a good option for people who have problems with vision or dexterity.

When Hearing Aids Aren't Enough

Hearing aids may not necessarily be the last or final option for a person with hearing loss. Some losses can be so severe that hearing aids are of little or no benefit regardless of how loudly they are set. The hearing aids are not of help because the ears can no longer process the sound they provide. Something different is needed.

A cochlear implant may be the answer for people whose hearing loss is beyond the range of hearing aids. This device restores hearing to severe or profoundly hearing-impaired people by electrically stimulating the underlying nerve cells in the inner ear. Part of the device is surgically implanted in the bone behind the ear. The other part of a cochlear implant is a speech processor that is worn behind the ear much like a BTE hearing aid. The speech processor picks up the sound. It codes and then transmits the sound to the internal part of the implant. The internal part supplies sound through tiny electrodes that extend into the inner ear. A cochlear implant does not restore normal hearing. It can, however, restore the awareness, pattern, pitch, and loudness of sound. It can often make possible speech understanding without lip reading.

Cochlear implants are not designed for people with mild or moderate hearing losses. These people do better with hearing aids. Even people with more severe losses may do better with hearing aids than they would with a cochlear implant. It is for this reason that a cochlear implant is not considered until a person has worn hearing aids and they have been shown to be of very limited or no benefit for the individual's hearing loss. While the technology incorporated within a cochlear implant is truly some of the most advanced and exotic available, it is not the appropriate device for the majority of people with hearing loss. Hearing aids are. Additionally, hearing aids are less expensive and do not require the invasive surgery of a cochlear implant.

Options and Add-Ons

Volume Control versus No Volume Control

The choice of whether or not to have a volume control on a hearing aid can be a little confusing. Years ago most hearing aids had a volume control. Today many of them—if not a majority—do not. This trend might imply that not having a volume control must be better. If this were the case, however, it would be difficult to explain why so many hearing aids are still being made with a volume control. What is the answer? Which choice is better?

The confusion here comes from asking the wrong question. The concern ought not be whether a hearing aid should or should not have adjustable volume. It should! The concern ought to be whether it will be the person who will adjust the volume or whether the hearing aid will be self-adjusting. Most of the older hearing aids were not very sophisticated compared to today's technology. They worked by making sounds a certain amount louder. No matter what fixed amount of amplification a person might choose, it would often be either too much or too little for what he or she was trying to hear. A volume control was absolutely essential. It let the hearing aid wearer adjust the hearing aids to the level that was optimal for the situation. Having a person adjust the hearing aids was necessary because the hearing aids could not do it.

With advances in electronics and miniaturization it has become possible to make hearing aids a little bit smarter. They can be programmed to recognize the difference between a soft whisper and a freight train. With this recognition it then becomes feasible for hearing aids to treat these situations differently. The whisper can be amplified until it is audible and the train kept from becoming too loud. Moment by moment the hearing aids decide how much sounds need to be amplified to keep them in a range that is both audible and comfortable. The hearing aids adjust the volume more than a person ever would or could.

The need to include a user-adjustable volume control depends largely on the sophistication of the hearing aid circuitry. The less sophisticated the circuitry, the more likely the wearer will need to step in and adjust the aids. The smarter the circuitry, the less need there will be for the wearer to adjust them. Many people buy relatively unsophisticated hearing aids because they cost less. They are willing to live with the trade-off of having to adjust the volume manually. This choice accounts for the majority of hearing aids with user-adjustable volume controls that are in use today. Even with the most sophisticated hearing aid circuitry, however, there is no guarantee that the hearing aids will always select a volume that a wearer will consider optimal. There might be times that a user would want to be able to have a little control. It is for this reason that some people who buy very sophisticated hearing aids still get a volume control even when they know that theoretically they should not need it. The volume control gives them a little more control over their situation.

Multiple Memories

A standard or optional feature on many programmable and digital hearing aids is the choice of multiple memories. By pressing a small button on the hearing aid or moving a switch, this feature allows a person to switch between programs tailored for different listening situations. The default program is usually set to help a person understand speech in quiet. The second program might be adjusted for listening in noisy environments. It might instead be adjusted to reproduce music faithfully. Most hearing aids with a multiple-memory option can accommodate two or three memory settings. The memories are programmed for a person's individual listening needs.

Directional Microphones

A common expectation of people buying hearing aids is that the hearing aids will allow them to focus in on whatever they would like to hear. The everyday application of this is that they expect to be able to hear and understand people talking regardless of background noise or other distracting factors. The people who have this expectation are usually disappointed to find that their hearing aids tend to amplify all of the sounds around them, not just what they wish to hear. As has been discussed, even if it were possible to filter out unwanted sounds, it is not possible for the hearing aids to always know which sounds a person would or would not want filtered out. A more practical solution is to focus on sound from one area and to exclude sound from everywhere else. The key to making this work is to focus on where, rather than on what, a person needs to hear.

Most hearing aids use an omni-directional microphone. This kind of microphone picks up sounds equally from all directions. You may want to hear the person directly across from you, but with an omni-directional microphone you hear not only that person, but also everything beside and behind you. This can be a real problem if people speaking surround you, as happens at a restaurant or at a party. Even though you may hear the speaker, there may be too much else going on for you to distinguish their speech from all the surrounding sound.

A directional microphone is the hearing aid option that would allow a person to focus in on where a person would like to hear. In contrast to an omni-directional microphone, a directional microphone primarily picks up and amplifies sounds coming from the front. Surrounding sounds are amplified less so they are not as distracting. It lets a person focus in on what he or she wants to hear simply by facing the person speaking. Directional microphones remain an option even if a person has times that he or she would want to hear equally from all directions. Both a directional and an omni-directional microphone can be built into some hearing aids, allowing a person to switch back and forth between them, depending on their immediate hearing needs.

In short, directional microphones are a very effective but underappreciated way of focusing in on what a person would like to hear. Anyone who needs to hear in noisy situations should give serious consideration to this option. It is relatively inexpensive (compared to the cost of some hearing aid options) and readily available from many hearing aid manufacturers.

Telecoils

Another hearing aid option that merits serious consideration is a telecoil. As previously mentioned, this option allows a person to hold a telephone up to the ear without the risk of feedback. A person can flip a tiny switch that turns off the hearing aid microphone and turns on the telecoil. Rather than amplifying the sound coming from the phone, the telecoil processes the electromagnetic waves that radiate from the telephone earpiece. This lets a person hear on the phone just as well, if not better, than if he or she were using the hearing aid microphone. An added benefit is that surrounding sounds that might compete with what a person is trying to hear are blocked because the microphone is turned off.

People who use a telecoil typically get one for only the ear they use on the phone. They save the expense of a second one since it would likely go unused. If, however, a person wishes to use his or her hearing aids with the assistive listening systems available at many theaters, public buildings, tourist attractions, and so forth, then a telecoil in each hearing aid would be better than having just one. This secondary use of telecoils is unfortunately underappreciated and underused.

One new advance is a switchless telecoil that activates itself when a person uses the phone. This convenient option is currently available on only a few high-end hearing aids. Hopefully this new option will gain wider availability with time.

Remote Control

A few programmable and digital hearing aids offer the option of a remote control. The majority of these remotes are shaped like a small calculator but others are shaped to resemble a wristwatch or a fountain pen. The goal is to make it possible or easier to change hearing aid settings. Completely-in-the-canal (CIC) hearing aids are so small that there is not usually room to include a volume control or button to change programs. If this were possible, the aid sits too far in the ear to use these kinds of controls easily. Having a remote control is a practical alternative. A remote control can also be helpful with larger hearing aids. Even a large hearing aid can become very cluttered and difficult to work if a person takes advantage of several hearing aid options. A person might bump the telecoil switch while trying to adjust the volume or turn up the volume while trying to change to a quieter program. Using a remote simplifies this process. It can also be helpful for people with limited dexterity who want to be able to take advantage of some of these options.

My experience with remote-control hearing aids has been that people either strongly like them or strongly dislike them. There are few people who are undecided regarding this option. They either like the ease of control made possible by the remote or dislike having to remember and fuss with it.

Windscreen

A windscreen covering the hearing aid microphone was previously discussed as a useful option for reducing wind noise. It should be considered a must for people who spend a lot of time outdoors. There is not usually an added charge for including a windscreen as long as it is ordered when the hearing aid is made. A person just has to remember to ask for it.

Making a Choice

Trial Periods

Audiologists and hearing instrument specialists are required by law in the United States to sell their hearing aids with the guarantee that they may be returned within thirty days for a refund (minus a trial fee) if a person is unsatisfied for any reason. Surprisingly, few people are aware of this option even though it is available to everyone. Furthermore, not all hearing aid fitters bother to explain the trial process to a potential hearing aid buyer. The terms of the trial are often buried in the fine print of the hearing aid sales agreement. The trial fee should be no more than about 10 percent of the total purchase price. A few hearing aid fitters do not charge anything if a hearing aid is returned. These professionals are the exception, however, rather than the rule. Anyone considering the purchase of hearing aids should talk with their hearing instrument specialist or audiologist to be sure he or she understands the return policy.

One reason that some audiologists and hearing instrument specialists are reluctant to discuss the option of trying hearing aids is that they do not want to create a self-fulfilling prophecy. They feel that a person who plans to try hearing aids will do only that. They will try, but not keep them. This is considered different from the person who plans to purchase hearing aids to compensate for a hearing loss. In the first case the act of trying hearing aids fulfilled the person's goal. In the second case hearing better fulfilled the goal. Audiologists and hearing instrument specialists that minimize their discussion of a hearing aid trial are often only acting to ensure that the appropriate goal in buying hearing aids is kept in mind. If one of their patients is dissatisfied at the end of the trial period, the hearing aid professional then discusses the option to return the hearing aids or to try different ones. Of course, a few that fail to mention the trial are scoundrels who are only interested in hearing aid sales. Being aware of your rights can protect you from these few.

If a person has tried hearing aids with the proper intent and still does not feel he or she hears better, the process of having tried them should not necessarily be viewed as a failure. Much can be learned by determining why this initial hearing aid fitting was considered unsuccessful. There are often alternative circuitry options or programming possibilities that may still work very well. The specific problems encountered with the first set of hearing aids serves as the guide for selecting alternatives.

If, however, you give hearing aids a serious try and remain dissatisfied or do not think you will wear them, you should return the hearing aids and pay only the trial fee.

More Expensive Is Not Always More Beneficial

If the three categories of hearing aids (analog, programmable, and digital) were sold in a department store, they would likely be promoted as good, better, and best. In many ways this would be a fair representation of their technological sophistication and the benefits they can provide. Not surprisingly, their prices reflect this progression. Some individuals with hearing loss will insist on buying the "best" hearing aids regardless of the cost. Instead, it may be a son that feels his father deserves the best or a husband insisting that nothing is too good for his wife. Other more budget-minded individuals may wonder whether the more-expensive hearing aids are really worth the higher cost.

The mistake that is often made in buying hearing aids is to assume that better or more-advanced technology must also mean more beneficial. This is not always the case. A person with a very mild hearing loss who needs only a little bit of increased volume may find that he or she does very well with analog hearing aids. The sound would be clear, the hearing aids would let the person hear soft sounds and, because there is only a modest increase in gain, loud sounds may not be too loud. Similarly, a person with a larger hearing loss may do well with this less-expensive circuitry if he or she has relatively easy listening demands. Directional microphones may have no added benefit for a person who is homebound and does not need to hear in noisy situations. Paying extra for a hearing aid with multiple memories will not provide extra benefit if a person does not have the dexterity to work the switch. If most of what needs to be heard takes place in one-on-one situations and there is limited surrounding noise, buying more-expensive hearing aids may not necessarily provide an increased benefit over conventional hearing aids.

Nevertheless, paying for added technological sophistication can have clear benefits. A digital aid with multiple channels and bands can better compensate when a person's hearing thresholds or sensitivity to loud sounds varies dramatically from one frequency to another. A hearing aid with multiple memories can offer a distinct advantage for a person who needs to hear in changing listening environments.

The question that a person needs to ask is: "With my particular hearing loss, listening demands, and lifestyle, what added benefit would I get from programmable or digital hearing aids over what would be obtained with traditional analog aids?" A similar question can be asked regarding hearing aid options or add-ons. If there is not an extra benefit in buying more-expensive hearing aids or hearing aid features, then a person can buy ones that are more basic.

One versus Two Hearing Aids

Prospective hearing aid wearers occasionally ask me if they really need two hearing aids or if one would be sufficient. It is true that they would hear better with one hearing aid than with no hearing aid. They would usually hear better, however, with two hearing aids. People are not born with one ear and a spare. The two ears are meant to be used together.

The advantages of two hearing aids have already been discussed. They include improved localization, better hearing in noise, elimination of the head shadow effect, and prevention of auditory deprivation. These advantages are sacrificed with the use of only one hearing aid. This is true regardless of the sophistication of the hearing aid chosen.

Selecting a Hearing Aid Manufacturer

One of the first questions hearing aid candidates have is "What brand of hearing aids should I buy?" The answer is that any quality hearing aid will be better than no hearing aid. Perhaps as much as 90 to 95 percent of the hearing improvement experienced by a hearing aid user is gained regardless of the brand chosen. People notice a clear improvement with hearing aids over how they hear without. Individual brands do make a difference, but the difference is more subtle and may not always be as noticeable.

Manufacturers advertise extensively to make their brand name and product lines familiar to us, but the hearing aids available from one manufacturer may not always be all that different from what is offered by their competitors. There may also be similarities between available add-ons. A single-channel programmable hearing aid from one manufacturer may perform very much like a similar aid from another manufacturer. A telecoil from two different companies may perform similarly. This is not to say, however, that there are no differences between brands. A two-channel digital hearing aid made by one manufacturer may divide each channel into separate bands that allow added signal processing while one made by another manufacturer may not have this extra adjustability. One manufacturer may include two programmable memories on a digital aid while a competitor may include three on a similar product. Some of these differences are proprietary while others are due to philosophy or cost concerns.

A selected, alphabetical list of established manufacturers that sell a wide range of hearing aids is shown in box 7.1. The key to selecting hearing aids is often not so much deciding between one of these or another brand as in selecting the most appropriate hearing aids from within a particular brand. It might instead involve finding a manufacturer that offers the combination of options that a person would want on a specific hearing aid. A person can decide what circuitry and options he or she wants in a hearing aid and select it from one manufacturer's product line or, if necessary, go in search of another company that makes it.

Utilizing Hearing Aid Professionals

Audiologists and hearing instrument specialists are the professionals who can help a person to select the hearing aid style, circuitry, and options that will best meet his or her needs. These professionals know what hearing aid options are likely to be beneficial for a person's hearing loss and lifestyle. They are also the ones who know which combinations of options are available from which manufacturer. A person does not have to make all of the hearing aid choices by him- or herself.

A Few Choices

Myrna Brock was a seventy-two-year-old widow who lived by herself. Although she was in good health and drove her own car, she was

---

Box 7.1 Ten Established Hearing Aid Manufacturers

1. Beltone	5. Phonak	8. Starkey
2. GN ReSound	6. Siemens	9. Unitron
3. Miracle Ear	7. Sonic	10. Widex
4. Oticon	Innovations	

---

not very active outside the house. She loved to talk with her sisters on the phone but was having increasing difficulty understanding them. She also reported problems hearing her children and grandchildren when they visited. Mrs. Brock was highly motivated to hear but was on a fixed income that she feared would limit her options. She could afford only one hearing aid but wanted to buy the most-sophisticated aid that was within her price range. This would have been a single-channel programmable hearing aid. In her situation she would likely do as well with a basic analog hearing aid, and this choice would allow her to add a telecoil and stay within her budget. She chose this option for her right ear since she was right-handed and also used this ear on the phone. The aid came standard with a volume control that she could adjust. The telecoil was the only added option. She felt the hearing aid helped significantly and especially enjoyed her renewed ability to hear on the phone.

Terry Unger was a forty-three-year-old account executive for a radio station. He suffered from a hereditary hearing loss that left him with a significant hearing deficit except at one narrow range of frequencies where he had normal hearing. The loss caused him listening difficulties at work and at home. He had unsuccessfully tried analog hearing aids in the past. The aids he tried were unable to amplify only the pitches where he had his loss. They overpowered him because some of the amplified sounds always crossed over into his good hearing range. After a discussion of the available options Mr. Unger agreed to try binaural digital hearing aids. The aids had multiple channels that could be adjusted independently. The added adjustability of the multiple channels made it possible to amplify sounds at only those frequencies where he had a hearing loss. This not only allowed him to hear, but also to hear comfortably. They also had two memory settings. His first memory program was adjusted for listening to speech in quiet environments. The second memory was adjusted for noisy environments. He found that having a second memory helped, but that he still had difficulty hearing in loud restaurants. Despite this limitation, Mr. Unger was happy with the overall result.

Susan Beck was a fifty-nine-year-old widow. She worked full-time in the housewares department of a large department store.

Although she felt her hearing was not a problem in most situations, she was experiencing difficulty understanding at work. She had delayed having an evaluation because she feared that it would lead to a hearing aid that she could not afford. She said she knew how much they cost because her husband's insurance had bought him two hearing aids shortly before his death. Mrs. Beck's evaluation confirmed her suspicion of a hearing loss. Hearing aids were recommended. Her employer's insurance plan did not provide hearing aid benefits. The benefits that would have been available through her husband's insurance were lost when the company he had worked for went bankrupt. Fortunately, her husband had programmable behind-the-ear hearing aids that could be reprogrammed to compensate for her hearing loss. All that was needed was to make earmolds that would fit her ears. This was done at a minimal cost that she could easily afford. She was thrilled with the result.

Albert Black was a ninety-two-year-old nursing home resident who suffered from the early stages of Alzheimer's disease. His hearing loss had been caused by years of noise exposure in a steel mill. His health insurance had bought him hearing aids but he had lost them. Fortunately, the aids came with a warranty against loss so he was able to get a new set. These were also lost. His daughter reported that he wore the hearing aids whenever he had a visitor and that they were a great help. He needed something to help him hear, but he did not have the money to keep buying hearing aids now that he had exhausted his insurance. The solution was a personal amplifier purchased at a local electronics store. It allowed him to hear and was affordable enough to replace if lost. Because of its larger size, it was also easier for the workers at the nursing home to find when it did get mislaid.

The stories of Mrs. Brock, Mr. Unger, Mrs. Beck, and Mr. Black serve to illustrate that there is no universal best hearing aid solution. The best solution is determined on an individual basis. Selection of specific hearing aids and hearing aid options should be based on a person's own hearing loss, lifestyle, and listening needs. This will provide a far superior result to selecting hearing aids based only on brand name or price.

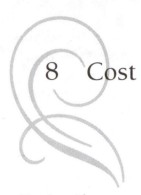

8   Cost

Hearing aids are a major expense. It should be no surprise that people would worry about how to pay for them or worry if they are worth the cost. People are also hesitant to spend money on hearing aids because they are not always certain that they will help. Some of the most sensible reasons for putting off or not buying hearing aids are related to cost. Even people who desperately need and clearly want hearing aids can be stopped here. The very group that needs them most—seniors—often have a limited income and usually not very good insurance. The situation for others is not necessarily any better.

This chapter examines the issue of cost. Discussed first is why hearing aids are expensive and what they typically cost. Incidental hearing aid expenses are discussed next. Presented last are insurance and other issues related to affording hearing aids.

Hearing Aid Prices

Reasons for the Cost

At a time when consumer electronics prices are at an all-time low, the price of hearing aids continues to increase. Calculators, radios, compact disc players, video cassette recorders, televisions, and computers are all at prices so low it would have been unthinkable a few years ago. The cost of the electronic components has gone down as well as the manufacturing cost. In this kind of economic atmosphere, a person shopping for hearing aids is likely to be in store for a serious case of sticker shock. Basic hearing aid prices have certainly not gone down over the past few years, and some of the newer models cost two to three times as much as their predecessors. How could anyone conclude that hearing aids are not too expensive?

There's a good explanation why hearing aids are so expensive, though this might not make your choice any easier. First, it is important to realize that most hearing aids are custom-made devices. A manufacturer cannot simply create and sell a million identical hearing aids in the same way they would television sets. The shape of a hearing aid has to fit the person's ear exactly and the electronics inside need to be those that will best compensate for an individual's particular hearing loss. The amount of customization needed makes the whole process labor intensive and drives up the cost of manufacture and fitting.

Manufacturers will claim that, as with pharmaceuticals, the high prices are necessary to recover research and development costs. Developing hearing aid technology is no different. Staying on the cutting edge of what is technologically possible drives up the cost enormously. The situation is in some ways like buying generic versus brand-name medication. The generic is almost always cheaper because all a pharmaceutical company has to do is make it. They did not have to pay to invent it. Furthermore, unlike pharmaceuticals that may continue to be sold long after research and development costs have been recovered, most hearing aids developed ten or twenty years ago have been replaced with newer models and are unavailable.

With advances in digital technology, there may come a day in the not-too-distant future where the price of hearing aids declines. This is because digital hearing aids are much like little computers that can be programmed in a variety of ways. The technology is approaching an "open platform" hearing aid design that could be programmed for any hearing loss. This would eliminate the need to constantly reinvent the hearing aid hardware. The price would drop because everyone would be able to use the same hearing aid circuitry. It is yet to be seen, however, whether this will happen or whether the research monies will go toward the development of better programming strategies for hearing aids or into CEO pockets.

Average Hearing Aid Prices

Although custom-made hearing aids can be very expensive, they aren't necessarily as expensive as you think. They range in cost from

$800 to $3,000 each. This price often includes the fitting fee and related professional services. It may also include free batteries for a set
period of time or for the life of the hearing aid. With the wide difference in price, however, you get a difference in size and sophistication. An $800 hearing aid will likely be one of the larger sizes and
have an analog amplifier. A $3,000 aid is likely to be a digital CIC or
a larger digital aid with all the bells and whistles. The average 2001
hearing aid prices reported from the *Hearing Journal*'s annual hearing instrument dispenser survey (Kirkwood 2002) are shown in box
8.1. These results serve as a good reference for judging the reason-
ableness of a quoted hearing aid price. They also illustrate the impact of hearing aid size and technology on price. Someone wanting
the smallest hearing aid possible within a particular class of aid (e.g.,
analog or digital) may have to pay as much as $500 extra for this cos-
metic advantage. Upgrading to a digital circuit may add $1,500 to
the price. The results also illustrate that there can be different prices
between basic and high-end products within a particular class. This
is clearly shown for programmable aids. Although not documented
in these results, this within-class variance can be even greater for
digital hearing aids.

Disposable Hearing Aid Prices

The cost of disposable hearing aids is about one dollar per day. Fitting fees and professional services are not included in this price. The
original disposable aids cost about $40 each and were estimated to last
forty days if used ten hours per day. A newer digital version costs $79

Box 8.1 Average 2001 Hearing Aid Prices

	BTE	ITE	Canal	CIC
Standard Analog Hearing Aid	$818	$830	$990	$1,326
Basic Programmable Aid	$1,179	$1,197	$1,372	$1,663
High-End Programmable Aid	$1,563	$1,604	$1,764	$2,001
Digital Aid	$2,235	$2,317	$2,474	$2,734

Source: D. H. Kirkwood, "Although Opinions Vary, Survey Finds Many Concerned by Consolidation of Dispensing," *Hearing Journal* 55, 3 (2002).

---

each and is estimated to last seventy days based on this same usage. Additional hours of use per day would shorten the life of each proportionally.

Disposable hearing aids are attractive because they do not require the large up-front costs of custom hearing aids. Over the long term, however, they are not necessarily less expensive than a custom aid. The real trade-off for the lower up-front costs are all of the advantages that come with having an aid that is individually customized to an ear.

Mail-Order Hearing Aid Prices

Although hearing healthcare professionals usually recommend against mail-order hearing aids, there is a large financial incentive for people to try them. The average cost of a mail-order hearing aid is typically $200 to $300 plus shipping. Even the most expensive rarely exceed one-half the price of a regular aid. This would be a bargain if these truly were equivalent to custom-made hearing aids. The reality is that they are miniature amplifiers. They may provide some benefit, but they are not usually individually customized for a person's hearing loss or for the size and shape of an individual's ear canal. The result can be a benefit that is equivalent to their lower cost. Nevertheless, they can help at least some and have a money-back guarantee for anyone who is dissatisfied.

Personal Amplifiers

A personal amplifier can be purchased for as little as $25 from an electronics store. It requires headphones that may cost an additional $7 to $10 if you do not already own a set from a personal stereo. More sophisticated personal amplifiers can be purchased from a hearing instrument specialist or audiologist. These can cost from $75 to $200 depending on the model and markup. Even the least expensive of these purchased from an electronics store generally work well to make sounds louder. The more-expensive models from hearing professionals may have less distortion at high volumes or have added features such as a remote microphone for listening to the television.

The Cost of Modifying Used or Donated Hearing Aids

Although audiologists and hearing instrument specialists do not typically sell used hearing aids, they can often modify a hearing aid that was made for one person to work for another. Someone who was left a hearing aid by a deceased friend or relative most often makes this request. Rather than buy new, the person would prefer to use the one he or she inherited. A BTE hearing aid may only need a new earmold to comfortably fit a new user. This could cost as little as $50. It is necessary to rebuild an ITE, canal, or CIC aid into a custom-fit plastic shell before a new user can comfortably wear it. The $250 to $300 this can cost is more than that required to adapt a BTE aid, but much less than purchasing a new hearing aid. There can, however, be additional reprogramming, adjustment, or professional fees. Getting a new earmold for a BTE aid is almost always a good investment as long as the BTE aid works well and is an appropriate one for the hearing loss. Rebuilding a fairly new (one to five years old) ITE, canal, or CIC aid can also be a good investment. There is the risk in rebuilding an older aid that it might not last long enough to justify the expense of modification.

Incidental Expenses

Batteries

Batteries are a person's most obvious incidental expense from hearing aids. All hearing aids use a battery. Each battery lasts about two weeks in the average hearing aid. Powerful hearing aids designed for severe losses or hearing aids with exotic circuitry may need more power and drain batteries faster. Hearing aids designed for mild hearing losses use less power and may have a longer battery life. A hearing aid user can easily change the battery without help. No special tools or training are required.

Batteries are available from the people who sell hearing aids and also from drugstores, discount stores, electronics stores, and other stores that sell specialty batteries. They are sold in packs of three, four, six, eight, and sixteen. The cost is generally $1.00 to $1.50 per battery when purchased from hearing aid centers or department stores. Many hearing aid centers offer a discount if the batteries are purchased in bulk. Larger bulk discounts can often be found on the Internet.

Although some people see batteries as a large reoccurring expense, you are likely to spend more money on gasoline going to and from the store to get batteries than on buying the individual batteries themselves. Because of the perception that batteries are very expensive, some audiologists and hearing instrument specialists include free batteries for the lifetime of any hearing aid they sell. Ask your audiologist if this is an option if you are concerned about this cost. Beware, however, this service may in turn result in a slightly higher price for the hearing aids.

One alternative to replacing the battery every couple of weeks is to buy a hearing aid with a rechargeable battery. These hearing aids are often advertised as not needing conventional batteries. They still use a battery, however, that will eventually wear out and need to be replaced after being recharged a certain number of times. The disadvantage to a rechargeable hearing aid is that it needs to be charged each night. If you forget, you may be without a hearing aid the next day.

Loss and Damage

Worry about losing hearing aids is a common and valid concern. As hearing aids get smaller and smaller, they become easier to misplace. They can get knocked onto the floor, brushed into the garbage, left at the hairdresser's, or mislaid in one of a million other ways. If not lost, hearing aids can be dropped, sat on, or crushed. Because of the high cost, hearing aids are definitely something a person would not want to lose, break, or have to pay to replace. To reduce this concern, many people prefer to commit to the incidental expense of damage and loss insurance for their hearing aids.

The risk of loss is sometimes overestimated. Most hearing aid users do not lose their hearing aids. Nevertheless, new hearing aid users may worry that the hearing aids will fall out of their ears and become lost. This almost never happens. Hearing aids are designed to fit the exact shape of the ear and usually stay in place very well. In the rare case where a hearing aid might fall out, a person could immediately feel that it is gone and pick it up before it becomes lost. It is usually when people take the hearing aids out of their ears and set them down in an unusual place that they become lost. They lose the hearing aids because they are not wearing them. It gives added meaning to the old adage "use it or lose it." Developing a habit with the hearing aids can prevent this.

A few individuals have the unfounded fear that an aid will become lost in another way. They fear that the hearing aid will go so far down into the ear canal that it will get stuck and be irremovable. A few others fear that the hearing aid will go down their ear canal and become lost somewhere in their head. This is simply not the case. While it might be theoretically possible for a hearing aid to get stuck in the ear, the shape of the ear makes this highly unlikely. If for some reason a person could not remove his or her hearing aid, an audiologist or physician most certainly could. The other idea that a hearing aid would fall into the ear canal and get lost in the head is anatomically impossible because the eardrum acts as a barrier to prevent the aid from going any further. This is not something that needs to be insured against.

Anyone who has never misplaced their car keys, lost expensive jewelry, or sat on their eyeglasses might not be interested in insuring their hearing aids. For everyone else, this can make financial sense and provide peace of mind. There may not be a great chance of loss or damage, but even one occurrence can be costly. Although hearing aids come with a warranty that gives protection against their not working properly, many do not include coverage for physical damage or loss. If there is a warranty against damage and loss, it does not usually extend longer than one year after purchase. Because of this, hearing aid loss and damage insurance should be a consideration. This kind of insurance can usually be purchased from an audiologist or hearing instrument specialist for $50 to $150 per year, depending on the make and model of hearing aid. Hearing aids may also be covered under some homeowner's and renter's insurance policies.

Repairs

The need for hearing aid repairs can be another incidental expense. While a person may get many years of service from a hearing aid without a major problem, it is not uncommon to need at least one or two major repairs along the way. This might be due to a receiver damaged by earwax, a microphone damaged by moisture, or some component that has just worn out. Your audiologist or hearing instrument specialist will usually send the hearing aid back to the manufacturer if a major repair is required. The standard hearing aid repair fee ranges from $130 to $200. The cost may be more than this in extreme cases, but manufacturers usually stick to their standard repair rate. To avoid the risk of repair fees, some people prefer to buy an extended warranty for their hearing aids. The cost of this can range from $100 to $200 per year, depending on the brand, style, and age of the hearing aid. Although buying this insurance can provide peace of mind, the above numbers illustrate that it is not always the best financial choice.

Minor repairs can often be performed by your audiologist or hearing instrument specialist. These repairs might include things like unplugging a receiver opening that is plugged by wax, replacing a broken battery door, cleaning corroded battery contacts, replacing old tubing on a BTE earmold, and so on. Some audiologists and hearing instrument specialists perform these minor repairs at no charge for the life of any hearing aid they sell. Others charge an office visit or minor repair fee. Don't be shy about asking your audiologist or hearing instrument specialist about his or her policy for these minor repairs.

Affording Hearing Aids

Health Insurance

The hearing aid industry grew up apart from medicine. Hearing aids were originally sold only by hearing aid dealers. Physicians and audiologists would refer to these dealers, but did not sell hearing aids themselves. To do so was considered a conflict of interest. The attitudes about this have changed with time. Audiologists are now at the forefront of hearing aid dispensing and ear, nose, and throat physicians often employ dispensing audiologists to provide a fuller range of care within their practice. The fact that it was not medical professionals who initially sold hearing aids, however, helped to set the stage for hearing aids to be considered a nonmedical device that was exempt from insurance coverage. Insurance will usually pay for an ear surgery or a cochlear implant, but not for hearing aids. The majority of insurance carriers do not include hearing aids as a covered benefit for their policyholders. In fact, some insurance companies go out of their way to make it clear that they do not ever pay for hearing aids. At the time of this writing, Medicare is one of these. There have been movements over the years to try to mandate hearing aid coverage, but these have generally failed due to cost constraints. To remain competitive, companies are often forced to purchase the least-expensive health insurance available for their employees. One of the ways this is obtained is by eliminating coverage for all but major medical problems. This effectively excludes hearing aids. Many government programs such as Medicare do not budget the money to cover hearing aids.

Hearing aids are, however, a covered benefit for many of the people who work in auto plants, steel mills, and other occupations where there is a strong labor union that fights for a higher level of insurance benefits. A few private insurance carriers also cover hearing aids to some extent, but one has to read the fine print carefully to know the details. Anyone with a hearing loss who is shopping for health insurance should consider each policy's hearing aid benefits when comparing the overall value of the policy. Hearing aid benefits are not all created equally.

The insurance plans that do provide hearing aid benefits will usually pay a predetermined amount toward one or two hearing aids every three or four years. They typically define this amount as being coverage for a standard hearing aid. The amount paid by an insurance company to the hearing aid fitter, however, may not be as much as the fitter normally charges for even a basic analog aid. It is often less than the fitter pays for a programmable or digital aid. Sometimes it is much less. This places severe limits on the hearing aid styles and circuitry that can be selected without the purchaser having to pay the balance. This presents a dilemma and a choice. People with difficult listening needs who purchase only what their insurance will cover may be dissatisfied with the hearing result. People who instead purchase a sophisticated hearing aid may find that they are left with a large bill despite having insurance coverage. Fitters who agree to accept only what an insurance company will pay without balance billing a patient are generally making the choice for the patient.

Payment on Delivery

Lack of insurance coverage can make affording hearing aids difficult. Those individuals who are not totally disheartened at discovering they are responsible for the cost of the hearing aids often do become disheartened when they discover that most audiologists or hearing instrument specialists want the total purchase price up front. The money serves as a security deposit. It is returned (minus a trial fee) if a person decides not to keep the hearing aids. A few of the smaller hearing aid practices do trust their patients to try hearing aids with little or no deposit. Even these trusting hearing aid fitters, however, frequently switch to a policy that requires a full security deposit if they experience too many instances where they do not receive payment for the hearing instruments they dispense or for their professional services.

Financing is another sticking point. Many people feel they need to spread out the cost of hearing aids over time. People buy cars this way and feel the process should be as easy for hearing aids. The problem is that unlike car dealers, most of the centers that dispense hearing aids are small enterprises that cannot afford to have a loan officer on staff. They also cannot afford to front the money themselves. They do, however, sometimes work with independent finance companies. This allows a person to buy hearing aids with little money up front as long as a person has a good credit history and is willing to make payments to this separate firm. Hearing aid centers also usually take credit cards.

Being Unemployed and Affording Hearing Aids

One of the times that people most need hearing aids may be one of the most difficult times to obtain help. This is when a person is unemployed and trying to get a job. If a person had been fortunate enough to have insurance coverage for hearing aids with his or her former job, these benefits would have been lost now that he or she is unemployed. While some individuals might finance this kind of expense, getting a loan may not be possible without a job. Even if a person has enough money to purchase hearing aids, it may be wiser to hold off making this investment because it is uncertain how long the person will remain unemployed. Although government programs and charitable organizations may provide hearing aids to the most destitute of individuals, they may not have the resources to help everyone in this situation. What is needed is a low-cost alternative to get people by at least in the short-run.

The often-overlooked alternative for the unemployed or for people with a temporary cash-flow problem is to purchase disposable hearing aids. These can be purchased for a minimal up-front cost and be replaced only as needed or as can be afforded. They may not always be as comfortable in the ear or as finely tuned to a specific hearing loss as a custom-made hearing aid, but they can still help a person to hear. Once a person finds a job or resolves the cash-flow problem, he or she could either continue to use disposable hearing aids or purchase ones that are custom made.

Dire Need

There are people who really need hearing aids, but do not have the money to pay for them. For this last group there is limited help available from charitable organizations and even some hearing aid manufacturers. They will either donate hearing aids or sell them at a greatly reduced price when there is clear proof of financial need. An ear doctor, audiologist, or hearing instrument specialist should be able to recommend who in your area might be able to provide this help.

Concerns about Being Swindled

There is sometimes concern that the people who fit hearing aids may sell them when they are unnecessary or charge more than they should cost. People worry that hearing aid fitters may be dishonest. Regardless of this perception, the people who sell hearing aids are usually law-abiding. They have little choice. They are licensed by state hearing aid or audiology boards and have to comply with their rules of conduct and ethical guidelines. Any reported transgressions are investigated by the state licensing boards. Failure to follow the rules of appropriate conduct can result in the revocation of the professional's hearing aid or audiology license. Audiologists are not likely to risk throwing away all of the years they spent in school learning to become an audiologist simply to sell an extra hearing aid or two. Similarly, experienced hearing instrument specialists are unlikely to risk their career or hearing aid practice by misrepresenting themselves. As in any profession, there can always be a bad apple. These are an exception, however, rather than the rule. If you need hearing aids but are worried about buying them from a particular hearing aid center, contact the Better Business Bureau for a report about the center (see box 8.2). This would alert you if the center has a number of unresolved complaints.

Losing Disability Payments

A few people use their hearing loss as a source of income and fear that compensating for it with hearing aids will jeopardize this income. The money may be from disability insurance, a worker's compensation claim, a lawsuit, or a government program. The general rule for people who find themselves eligible for such monies is that the greater the hearing loss, the more money they are likely to receive. They know this and fear that by reducing their functional hearing loss with hearing aids, they will be reducing the amount of money received. They are concerned that by wearing hearing aids they would be cheated out of money to which they are rightfully entitled.

Fortunately, most programs designed to compensate persons for a hearing disability do not penalize them for trying to help them-

---

Box 8.2. Contacting the Better Business Bureau

The Better Business Bureau (BBB) offers reports on many businesses including hearing aid centers. Anyone wishing to get a report on a specific center will need the center's area code and phone number. A person can also file a complaint about a hearing aid center with the BBB and ask for their assistance in resolving a dispute. The BBB has a local phone number for most communities that can be found in your telephone business white pages. They can also be reached through their web site at http://www.bbb.org.

---

selves. The amount of hearing loss or handicap used to determine compensation is based on a person's hearing level without hearing aids. If a person gets hearing aids, the amount of hearing loss or handicap used to determine compensation is still based on the person's hearing level without the hearing aids. As a general rule, people who were eligible to receive money without hearing aids are still eligible for money with hearing aids.

For the few individuals who find themselves the exception to the above rule, there is a choice to be made. Is it better for a person to receive his or her full entitlement and not hear, or is it better to hear and forfeit or receive less entitlement? In this rare case, choosing the entitlement is much like a person selling a part of himself or herself. What is being sold is not just the chance to hear, but also the ability to participate easily in activities with others. It may not be like a person selling his or her soul, but it is a couple steps in that direction.

In Summary

Custom hearing aids are available in a range of prices—none of which are cheap. Even people with good insurance may need to pay extra for hearing aids that would be optimal for their hearing loss. Unfortunately, the majority of people have no hearing aid benefits. The entire hearing aid expense is out-of-pocket. While there are lower cost alternatives to custom hearing aids, these can also come with reduced benefit. People with hearing loss are something of a captive audience to hearing aid prices. You can buy less-sophisticated hearing aids at cheaper prices, but you cannot lower the price of a particular class of hearing aid. Miniaturization, sophisticated circuitry, and added options come at a higher price. Financial considerations may leave a person no choice but to buy the most basic hearing aid or even a non-custom alternative. Paying less for a cheaper hearing aid, however, does not make it a bargain if it does not match up well to your hearing loss. Fortunately, not everyone requires the most-sophisticated technology in order to hear well. Many people are pleasantly surprised to find that basic and less-costly hearing aids are what best fits their hearing loss and needs.

9 Rejoining the Hearing World

There is no one secret that will transform a person with hearing loss into a successful hearing aid user. Similarly, there is no one thing that family and friends can do to produce this transformation. A number of steps are required. The steps ultimately have to be taken by the person with hearing loss. Friends and family can, however, help the person along the way. The first part of this chapter describes each of these steps. The issues of importance for the person with hearing loss and also for his or her family and friends are explained at each step. The second part of the chapter provides sources for additional information.

Steps toward Successful Hearing Aid Use

Recognizing a Hearing Problem

Hearing loss usually begins long before a person or his or her family and friends suspect a problem. The process tends to be very gradual, so there is not any dramatic event that alerts anyone. Friends and family are often the first to suspect as they recognize more and more things they can hear that their friend or loved one cannot. For a person with hearing loss it is usually only after the loss has progressed to a degree that it clearly affects his or her quality of life that a problem is suspected.

A person may recognize his or her hearing problem without any outside help. This is most likely to happen when someone is very active and engaged with others. The person recognizes that friends and family are hearing things that he or she does not or that these others easily hear things he or she struggles with. Hearing loss affects quality of life because it limits a person's ability to participate in the activities he or she enjoys. A person who is active and engaged is bound to notice it.

In contrast, those persons who are not very engaged with others can be unaware of a fairly significant hearing loss. They may not realize that the only reason they can understand their family and close friends is that these people are yelling. They may be unaware that their neighbor is involuntarily listening to their television. They conclude that their hearing is fine and that the problem lies with other people who do not speak clearly. The pastor at church, the waitress in a restaurant, the teller at the bank, the paperboy collecting for the paper, and the barber or hairstylist doing their hair all must be mumbling. If only they would speak clearly like their friends and family members, there would not be a problem. The quality of these people's lives is affected by their hearing loss, but they may not be aware it is happening or of the extent to which it is happening.

A dose of tough love by family or friends can be the most effective approach to help a person recognize that he or she has a hearing loss or to recognize the extent to which it is affecting his or her life. Rather than speaking loudly to make it easier for a person with hearing loss, family and friends can speak at a normal volume. Rather than playing the television very loud, they can set it to a more normal level. Rather than shielding the person from situations that would be difficult, he or she can be thrown into these situations. Family and friends can take the person to a church social, a community meeting, or a play in a theater without an amplified sound system. They can encourage the person to spend more time talking with his or her grandchildren. They can find ways to demonstrate how the person's hearing loss is limiting what he or she can do. The intent is not to be mean. Rather, the goal is to put the person into realistic listening environments that serve to highlight the listening problem.

Confronting Hearing Aid Concerns

Previous chapters have discussed numerous hearing aid concerns. Left unaddressed, any one of these could prevent a person buying or successfully using hearing aids. These worries have to be dealt with because they can become the greatest obstacle to a person's hearing better. The majority of people with hearing loss never get past their hearing aid concerns to find out what could be done to help them hear better.

Knowledge is the key to helping people overcome these concerns. They discover that much of what they thought they knew about hearing aids was based on medical misconceptions. They find that many of their fears are unfounded or based on cases so unusual or extreme that these things would never apply to them. They find that the issues that might truly be a concern can be avoided or minimized so that they are less likely to stand in the way of their doing well with hearing aids. With a little knowledge, people begin to see that although hearing aids have limitations, these limitations do not prevent the hearing aids from being helpful.

Family and friends of a person with hearing loss often ask, "How do I overcome all of these concerns?" The answer is that by themselves, they cannot. Family and friends play a supportive role. Their role is to provide information and serve as a sounding board to help the person examine his or her concerns honestly.

Finding a Hearing Aid Professional

There are two general classes of people who sell hearing aids. The first of these are audiologists. They are university-trained professionals who perform, interpret, and counsel people regarding just about every kind of hearing- and ear-related test. They are trained to prescribe and fit hearing aids and other assistive hearing devices. They are also trained to help people to find ways in which to change their behavior or situation to make it easier for them to hear.

A master's degree in audiology from an accredited university has been the traditional training for an audiologist practicing clinically. An additional year of clinical practice under the supervision of an experienced audiologist is required before an audiologist can practice independently. The training to perform this work includes extensive coursework covering hearing problems, ear disorders, anatomy and physiology of the ear, speech and language pathology, acoustics, statistics, research, electronics, and other related areas. With even more education are audiologists who have a doctor of philosophy degree (Ph.D.) in audiology. This degree adds additional science and research training beyond the master's degree. Although some of these professionals practice clinically, the majority perform research and teach audiology in universities. Also having education beyond the master's degree are audiologists who have a clinical doctoral degree in audiology (Au.D.) Within a few years this clinical doctorate is expected to replace the master's degree as the minimum level of education required to enter the field.

The second group of people who sell hearing aids are hearing instrument specialists. This is the group people sometimes refer to as hearing aid dealers. Beginning hearing instrument specialists will often learn their trade from an experienced hearing instrument specialist. They may also obtain training from individual hearing aid manufacturers or from attending seminars. They do not, however, usually have the extensive university training of an audiologist and may not legally use the title audiologist.

Ideally, a person would want to select the best trained professional he or she can find to prescribe and fit his or her hearing aids. It is not, however, as simple as that. A person may live in a remote area and have few professionals to choose from. A person might instead have many professionals to choose from but have difficulty deciding which to select once he or she takes each professional's experience and personality into account. A person might opt to work with an experienced hearing instrument specialist who is caring and personable rather than with an audiologist he or she dislikes. A person might choose to work with an experienced audiologist having a master's degree than work with a Ph.D. or Au.D. who is fresh out of school. Finding a hearing aid professional that a person will be happy with is not just a matter of looking at the letters written after his or her name.

The Yellow Pages and advertisements can serve as a starting point for finding an audiologist or hearing instrument specialist in your area. Another approach would be to contact the American Academy of Audiology (http://www.audiology.com) or the American Speech-Language-Hearing Association (http://www.asha.org). The best way, however, for a person to find a good hearing aid professional is to talk with other people who have been to these professionals. If everyone agrees that an individual is professional and caring and that the services are reasonably priced compared to the competition, then the person has found his or her professional. If the hearing aid fitter is described as unprofessional and only interested in making a sale, then this professional is likely someone to avoid. A person should find the hearing aid professional that people would recommend to their friends and avoid the ones that people would never revisit.

Family and friends can have an important role in helping a person to find a good hearing aid professional. People with hearing loss are often uncomfortable talking about their loss with others. Because of this they are unlikely to seek out and talk with people who wear hearing aids. Left to their own devices, they will either do nothing or go to the audiologist or hearing instrument specialist who runs the largest advertisements in the newspaper. Family and friends can prevent this from happening. They can talk with people who wear hearing aids and find out which professionals are skilled and well liked. They can then direct their hearing-impaired friend or family member to this professional. If the person remains hesitant, friends or family members can get them together with a person who does well with his or her hearing aids and likes his or her hearing aid professional. This testimonial can then make the difference.

Ruling Out a Medical Problem

The initial consideration of most people with hearing loss is whether or not they would want to try hearing aids. This should not, however, be their only consideration. It should probably not even be the initial consideration. They should instead be asking a hearing professional the following questions:

1. Why do I have a hearing loss?
2. Can it be medically or surgically corrected?

Hearing aids should only be tried once these two questions have been addressed. The first question needs to be answered to be sure that a hearing loss is not a sign of a larger problem. It also needs to be answered to determine whether steps might be taken to prevent further loss of hearing. The reason for the second question is a little more obvious. A person should not have to compensate for a hearing loss that can be medically corrected. While most hearing losses cannot be eliminated medically, a few can. It is worthwhile for a person with hearing loss to find out if his or her loss is one of these few.

From a medical perspective, a person with hearing loss should start by seeing an ear doctor (otologist) or an ear, nose, and throat (ENT) doctor prior to going to a hearing aid center. If the hearing loss is something that can be medically treated or surgically corrected, these are the specialists who can do it. Federal law requires a person to have a medical evaluation prior to being fit with hearing aids or at least to be informed that a medical evaluation is in his or her best interest. Since most hearing losses are not medically correctable, however, the majority of people who have an evaluation from one of these very specialized doctors will still need to pursue hearing aids with an audiologist or hearing instrument specialist if they wish to hear better.

Because the odds lean toward a person with hearing loss ultimately needing to see an audiologist or hearing instrument specialist, many people choose to start with one of these specialists instead of a medical doctor. This does not mean that medical issues are not given consideration. Part of an audiologist's training includes his or her being able to recognize hearing losses that might be medically correctable. They are also trained to recognize when a patient's symptoms or test results would suggest the need for referral to a medical doctor. Even a hearing instrument specialist who may have no medical or audiological training is required to know the situations in which a medical referral would always be indicated.

The most common symptoms indicating the need to be seen by a medical doctor would include the following:

- Hearing that is worse in one ear than in the other.
- Drainage or discharge from an ear.
- An odor coming from the ear.
- Dizziness.
- Tinnitus (ringing) that is worse in one ear than in the other.
- Ear pain.
- A sudden loss of hearing.

Anyone experiencing these symptoms would be best served by first seeing an otologist or an ENT doctor. If a person having any one of these conditions were to start with an audiologist or hearing instrument specialist, he or she would still need to be seen by a physician to rule out a medical problem.

Dealing with a hearing loss is not only about hearing aids. It is about the hearing loss itself and about what the hearing loss might only be a symptom of. If a person has any of the above symptoms, he or she should see an ear doctor. If a family member or friend has any of the above symptoms, a person should recommend he or she see an ear doctor.

Selecting Hearing Aids

If you have done a good job of finding a hearing aid professional, then the task of selecting the most appropriate hearing aids is made easier. You do not have to know which hearing aid companies make a circuit that will compensate for your particular hearing loss. You do not have to know which companies can make a hearing aid small or narrow enough to fit into your ear canal if it is unusually shaped. It is not necessary for you to know which of the many possible hearing aid options would be most beneficial for your hearing loss and lifestyle. All of this is the job of the person fitting the hearing aids.

The average person considering hearing aids is typically concerned about three things: the size, the price, and whether he or she will have to adjust the volume. As a person with hearing loss, your job is to make sure your audiologist or hearing instrument specialist understands what you want. It is also your job to make sure the professional understands your hearing needs and greatest hearing difficulties. It is the job of the hearing aid professional to balance your wants and needs against what is likely to be the most beneficial hearing aid solution for you.

The role of family and friends in the hearing aid selection process is to make sure the person with hearing loss understands the recommendations of the hearing aid professional and that the hearing aid professional understands all of the person's hearing and lifestyle needs. Someone who lives alone and spends most of his or her time watching television may be very satisfied with only one relatively unsophisticated hearing aid. The choice of only one hearing aid would not be at all appropriate, however, if this same person volunteers part-time as a crossing guard for elementary schoolchildren. The person would need two hearing aids to be able to localize traffic sounds. Friends and family can point out these minor details that a person with hearing loss might fail to mention. This extra little bit of information can make all of the difference between a person who does well with his or her hearing aids and a person who does poorly because the wrong options were chosen.

Trying Hearing Aids

Once you have decided that hearing aids might help, the next step is to try them. As previously explained, hearing aids are purchased with the understanding that they may be returned within a set period of time (usually thirty days) if you are dissatisfied for any reason. If returned, there is a trial fee that should not exceed 10 percent of the cost of the hearing aids. The option of a trial does two things. It allows a person who is fairly sure that hearing aids would be of benefit to test out this belief with a minimum of risk. It also gives family, friends, and hearing aid professionals a chance to prove that a person could benefit from using hearing aids.

Although it is important that you be able to try hearing aids, you need to understand that this is not the end goal. Being able to hear better and participate more fully is the goal. The option of a hearing aid trial is only one small clause along the way. A person who sets out with the goal of trying hearing aids will often do only that.

Family and friends of a person with hearing loss also have a role to play during the trial process. One part of this role is to make sure the person understands that he or she can try hearing aids. This is not always known. The greater role for family and friends during the trial process, however, is to help the person recognize just how much the hearing aids do help. This is not always apparent to a person wearing hearing aids. A person who used to turn his or her television up very loud prior to hearing aids may not be aware that he or she is comfortably listening to it at a much lower level with the hearing aids. A family member commenting that he or she can now stand to be in the same room with the television serves to drive this point home. Friends and family can mention that they no longer have to yell to be understood. They can call attention to all of the other times the hearing aids make a clear difference. The primary role of family and friends during the trial process is to provide the person with enough feedback to make sure the person recognizes how much better he or she is doing with the hearing aids.

Successfully Using Hearing Aids

Although skeptics may be reluctant to believe it, there are people who love their hearing aids. The age, gender, amount of hearing loss, and listening situations for these successful hearing aid users may vary widely, but there are two common threads that connect them all. They consistently wear their hearing aids, and they have realistic goals regarding them.

The human brain is marvelously adaptable. A proof of this is that people get used to hearing with a hearing loss. Over time one person may adapt to hearing with a high-pitched hearing loss while another may get used to a low-pitched deficit or poor hearing across all pitches. People with these and other hearing losses are likely to say that their hearing sounds natural regardless of how unnatural the pattern of their loss. Adjusting to this, however, is not something that happened overnight.

Getting used to something different takes time. Those who consistently wear their hearing aids through most of their waking hours will adapt and become used to hearing with the aids. For them, it will be all of the things they do not hear when they take their hearing aids out that will seem unnatural. People cannot adapt to hearing aids by wearing them sporadically. This is a matter of constant change, and people do not usually do well with constant change. People who do well with hearing aids avoid this. They adjust to hearing with the hearing aids because this is what becomes normal for them.

The second attribute of successful hearing aid users is that they have realistic expectations regarding what the devices can and cannot do. The primary goal voiced by successful hearing aid users is that they want the hearing aids to help them hear better. This goal is readily achievable. People who have unachievable expectations such as the restoration of normal hearing turn into disappointed hearing aid users, or worse yet, hearing aid non-users.

Someone who wishes to do well with hearing aids will not succeed unless he or she wears them consistently and has realistic expectations. Friends and family of a person with hearing loss should make sure the person understands this. Friends and family should also examine their own expectations and take care that they do not become the source of expectations that are unattainable.

Listening Strategies

Hearing aids make it much easier for the average person with hearing loss to be able to hear and understand. They do not, however, restore perfect hearing. There will still be times even with hearing aids that a person may have difficulty hearing or understanding. This is true even for successful hearing aid users. This does not mean that hearing aids do not work, but rather, that there are limits to how much they can help. It is when these limits have been reached that a person may have to do a little bit extra to hear.

This extra is sometimes referred to as a listening strategy. A person develops a plan on how best to hear in a given situation. Getting close to the person speaking so that he or she will sound louder, being able to see the speaker so that lip reading is possible, and reducing background noise are the usual tools incorporated into one of these strategies. If a person cannot hear the softest spoken person at a business meeting, one strategy might be to sit next to him or her so the person will sound louder. A different strategy might be to sit directly across from the speaker. This aims the speaker's voice in the proper direction and makes lip reading possible. If a person cannot hear the minister at his or her church, possible strategies would be to sit directly in front of the pulpit or to sit near the speakers if the church has a public address system. When background noise is the problem, a person will do better if he or she can get close to the person talking. This will make the speaker louder in relation to the background noise. A different strategy might be to move to a quieter place where it is easier to hear or to eliminate the background noise by turning off or turning down a radio or television. Simply rearranging the furniture of a room can help. A person can put his or her favorite chair closest to what he or she wishes to hear and furthest from air-conditioner and furnace vents, the dishwasher, and other extraneous sources of noise. With just a little common sense most people can find ways to help themselves hear better. Even successful hearing aid wearers can benefit from occasionally rearranging their world.

Helpful Resources

Publications for People with Hearing Loss

People who are new to the topic of hearing loss or hearing aids sometimes look for a magazine or newsletter that will give them some background information. If they were already diagnosed with a hearing loss or already use hearing aids, they may look for a magazine that will keep them informed about any new advances that might benefit them.

Perhaps the best-known publication for people with hearing loss is *Hearing Health Magazine.* This magazine is written specifically for people with hearing loss. Contact information is listed below.

> Hearing Health Magazine
> P.O. Box 938
> 2989 Main St.
> Ingleside, Texas 78362
> 361-776-7240 Voice or TTY
> 361-776-3278 Fax
> web: http://www.hearinghealthmag.com
> email: ears2u@hearinghealthmag.com

Another good source of information is Self-Help for Hard of Hearing People (SHHH). They publish the magazine *Hearing Loss: The Journal of Self-Help for Hard of Hearing People.* Although the title makes this publication sound very technical, it is easy to read and loaded with useful information. While it is necessary to join their national organization to receive their magazine, it is well worth the cost. They also have regional groups. They can be contacted at

Self-Help for Hard of Hearing People, Inc.
7910 Woodmont Ave., Suite 1200
Bethesda, Maryland 20814
301-657-2248 Voice
301-657-2249 TTY
301-913-9413 Fax
web: http://www.shhh.org
email: national@shhh.org

Support Groups

There are organizations in addition to SHHH that offer self-help groups for people with hearing problems. The organizations also serve as a good source of information. A few of these organizations include

Alexander Graham Bell Association for the Deaf
3417 Volta Place, NW
Washington, D.C. 20007
202-337-5220
http://www.agbell.org

American Tinnitus Association
P.O. Box 5
Portland, Oregon 97207
800-634-8978
http://www.ata.org

League for the Hard of Hearing
71 W. 23rd Street
New York, New York 10010
917-305-7700
http://www.lhh.org

National Association for the Deaf
814 Thayer Ave.
Silver Spring, Maryland 20910

301-587-1788
http://www.nad.org

Information on the Internet

An often-overlooked source of information about hearing aids is the Internet. The primary reason for this oversight is the demographic of the average person with hearing loss. Although hearing loss can occur at any age, it occurs most frequently in old age. Many older individuals have never used a computer in the home or workplace. They may have gained some computer experience with the boom in personal computers, but, on average, they tend to be less computer savvy than people from other age groups. Senior citizens do have access to the Internet. If they do not own a computer, they usually have friends or relatives who would let them use their computer. Furthermore, most public libraries allow free access through their computers. Many seniors simply do not feel the need to use the Internet or recognize how useful it might be to them.

Anyone who is experienced with the Internet will attest to the fact that it can be a wonderful source of information. Regardless of what a person is interested in, there is probably information about it on the Internet. Hearing aids are no exception. A quick search for information about hearing aids using one of the major Internet search engines will list hundreds or thousands of potential sites. That is not to say that all of these sites will have information that will be helpful or even accurate. But with a little time and sorting, useful information is readily available. Some of the most useful links are

http://www.asha.org
http://www.ata.org
http://www.audiology.com
http://www.entnet.org
http://www.healthyhearing.com
http://www.hearinghealth.net
http://www.hear-it.org
http://www.nidcd.nih.gov

Another source of information on the Internet is available from listserve discussion groups. A person can read what others have to say about issues related to hearing loss and hearing aids and also ask questions and join in the discussion. A few of these listserves are

Alt.relationships.deaf-hearing
Alt.support.hearing-loss
Alt.support.tinnitus

One Final Comment about Hearing Loss and Hearing Aids

There is a solution for hearing loss. The solution is hearing aids! Is it a perfect solution? No. Is it a good solution? Yes! This solution is available now and can make a noticeable difference for the majority of people with hearing loss. Standing in the way of this help are a lack of information and many misguided concerns. As previously mentioned, fewer than one-fourth of the people who could be helped by hearing aids actually buy them. This leaves the remainder suffering needlessly. With only a little information and change in perspective, this need not be so.

Glossary

Analog Hearing Aid   A hearing aid that processes sound as a voltage. All of the older conventional hearing aids processed sound in this way.

Assistive Listening Device   A broad category of devices that are designed to help a person hear better in a specific situation. An amplified telephone, a public address system, or a set of wireless headphones that could bring sound right to a person would be examples.

Audiogram   The graph of a person's hearing.

Audiologist   A person university trained in the evaluation and rehabilitation of hearing problems. This includes hearing aids. An audiologist is essentially a hearing scientist.

Auditory Deprivation   This is a phenomenon in which the word understanding may decrease over time in the unaided ear of a person who wears only one hearing aid. The addition of a second hearing aid has been shown to reverse this trend in some but not all people who had worn only one hearing aid. The prevention of auditory deprivation is sometimes used as a reason to support the use of two hearing aids.

Auditory Rehabilitation   A general term that refers to teaching a hearing-impaired person to be able to make effective use of sound. Training in the use of hearing aids is often included in this process.

Auricle   The portion of the ear extending outward beyond the skull. Also called the pinna.

Automatic Gain Control (AGC)   Special circuitry within a hearing aid that self-adjusts the volume for the wearer.

Background Noise   Any sound we do not wish to hear at a particular moment. These unwanted sounds are an area of concern for most hearing aid users.

Behind-the-Ear (BTE) Hearing Aid   The battery and electronics in this form of hearing aid hang behind the ear. Sound is carried from the body of the aid through a small tube to an earmold that fits in the ear.

BICROS   This is a special version of a CROS hearing aid that is designed for a person with a partial hearing loss in one ear and a total hearing loss in the other. Part of the hearing aid is worn on the poorer hearing ear and transmits the sound across to a part on the better hearing ear. The part in the better hearing ear amplifies the sound from the better hearing side and the sound that is transmitted from the poorer hearing side. The sound is combined and put into the better hearing ear.

Binaural   Both ears.

Body Aid   The largest and most powerful of hearing aids. The electronics for the hearing aid and the battery that powers it are housed in a small case about the size of a pack of cigarettes that is worn somewhere on the body. The sound is carried through a small wire to an earpiece.

Bone Conduction Hearing Aid   A hearing aid that works by gently vibrating the skull rather than by putting sound in the ear. Bone conduction hearing aids are used for large conductive hearing losses that cannot be medically corrected.

Canal Aid   A hearing aid that fits entirely in the ear canal.

Cerumen   Earwax.

Cochlea   The portion of the inner ear that contains the structures that are responsible for hearing.

Cochlear Implant   An electronic device that is surgically implanted into the inner ear to restore sound to people with severe or profound deafness. A cochlear implant becomes an option if a person's hearing loss has progressed beyond the point where hearing aids are of benefit.

Completely-in-the-Canal (CIC) Hearing Aid   The smallest of the canal hearing aids.

Compression   A form of automatic gain control. As incoming sounds get louder and louder, the hearing aid adds less and less amplification so that the end result is not overpowering.

Concha Hearing Aid   Another name for an ITE or full-shell hearing aid.

Conventional Hearing Aid   A basic hearing aid that uses analog circuitry. This circuitry processes sound as a voltage in much the same way as is done by a radio. These tend to be relatively unsophisticated hearing aids that usually require the user to adjust the volume as needed.

CROS (contra lateral routing of signal) Hearing Aid   This kind of aid is designed for a person with normal hearing in one ear and a total hearing loss in the other. Part of the hearing aid is worn on the non-hearing ear and transmits the sound across to a part on the normal-hearing ear. By transmitting the sound to the opposite ear, the hearing aid effectively keeps a person's head from getting in the way of their normal-hearing ear. Sound coming toward the good ear can go into the ear naturally.

Custom Hearing Aids   Hearing aids that are individually made to fit the exact shape of a person's ears and to compensate for their individual hearing loss. The vast majority of hearing aids sold are custom fit.

Decibel (dB)   The units of loudness used to measure a person's hearing. The smaller the number, the better the hearing. Normal hearing thresholds range between zero to twenty decibels.

Digital Hearing Aid   A hearing aid that processes sound as numbers. It is like a miniature computer that can control or modify sound in almost an infinite number of ways simply by changing numbers within its program.

Directional Microphone   A special kind of microphone that can be built into a hearing aid. It lets a person focus in on sound coming from one direction rather than picking up sounds equally from all around.

Disposable Hearing Aid   A form of non-custom hearing aid that is mass-produced to be so inexpensive that it can be thrown away once its battery has worn out. This is the hearing aid equivalent of disposable contact lenses.

Distortion   The inexact reproduction of sound. As with any other high-fidelity device, there is a small amount of distortion that is normal in a hearing aid. A large amount of distortion, however, can be a sign of a malfunctioning hearing aid.

Dynamic Range   The difference between the softest sound a person can hear and the loudest sound that can be comfortably tolerated. Hearing aids are adjusted to keep their output within this range.

Ear Impression   A cast or mold made to determine the exact size and shape of an ear. The impression is used as the blueprint to make a custom-fitted hearing aid.

Earmold   The portion of a behind-the-ear hearing aid that fits into the ear. It is attached to the body of the aid by a clear tube.

Eustachian Tube   A small tube leading from the middle ear that allows the equalization of pressure between the middle ear and the outside world.

External Auditory Canal   The ear canal.

Eyeglass Hearing Aid   A style of hearing aid in which the working parts are built into a person's eyeglass frames. Similar to a BTE hearing aid, the sound is carried through a small clear tube to an earmold worn in one or both ears.

Feedback   The howling or whistling sound that is sometimes heard coming from a hearing aid. Feedback is caused by sound leaking around a hearing aid and into the microphone to be amplified again and again until all it can do is howl at its maximum loudness.

FM System   This is a form of assistive listening device that places a microphone next to a sound source and transmits the sound to the listener using FM radio signals. It effectively moves the listener's ear right up to the person talking. FM systems are often used in schools, lecture halls, and other settings where it is necessary to clearly hear a person some distance away.

Frequency   The pitch of a sound.

Full-Shell Hearing Aid   Another name for an ITE aid.

Half-Shell Hearing Aid   A style of hearing aid that is a little bit larger than a canal aid but smaller than an ITE aid.

Head Shadow Effect   This refers to the amount of sound that is blocked by a person's head before it can reach the opposite ear. This reduction of sound is an issue for people who only have hearing in one ear and people who choose to wear a hearing aid in only one ear.

Hearing Aid Style   The style is determined by the size and shape of a hearing aid. The most common styles ranging from smallest to largest are completely-in-the-canal (CIC), mini-canal, canal, half-shell, in-the-ear, behind-the-ear, and body aid.

Hearing Aid Trial   A provision in the hearing aid buying process that allows a person to return his or her hearing aids within a set period of time for a refund (minus a trial fee) if unsatisfied for any reason.

Hearing Instrument Specialist (HIS)   One of the groups of people who sell hearing aids. They are usually licensed by the individual states and required to pass a test for licensure to guarantee a minimal level of competency.

Hearing Threshold   The quietest level a person can hear at least half the time under ideal conditions.

Hertz (Hz)   The units in which the frequency of a sound is measured.

Incus   The centermost of the three middle ear bones. Also called the anvil.

Internal Feedback   A whistling that results when sound that is supposed to go into the ear goes instead directly to the microphone through a damaged hearing aid case and becomes amplified again and again. Internal feedback can also be due to an electronic fault in a hearing aid.

In-the-Canal (ITC) Hearing Aid   A style of hearing aid that fits entirely within the ear canal.

In-the-Ear (ITE) Hearing Aid   A general term used to refer to any hearing aid that fits entirely into the ear. It is also used to refer to the largest of the in-the-ear hearing aids that completely fills up the bowl-shaped portion of a person's ear. An ITE aid is also called a full-shell or concha aid.

Linear Hearing Aid   A hearing aid that increases the loudness of a sound by a set amount (10 percent, 20 percent, 30 percent, and so on) regardless of the starting point. This can result in soft sounds not being amplified enough to be heard and very loud sounds amplified so that they are uncomfortable. Most older hearing aids were linear.

Listening Strategy   A plan to hear better. The goal is to identify the situations where a person has the most difficulty hearing or has the most need to hear and then modify the situation in some way to gain a hearing advantage.

Malleus   The outermost of the three middle ear bones. Also called the hammer.

Masking   One sound covering up another. In regards to hearing aids, it usually refers to background sounds covering up what a person would like to hear or to the sound coming from the hearing aid helping to cover up a person's tinnitus.

Master Hearing Aid   A hearing aid with circuitry that can be adjusted to compensate for almost any hearing loss. Some of the older analog hearing aids were touted as being master hearing aids, but many of the newer digital aids come much closer to meeting this goal.

Mild Hearing Loss   A twenty- to forty-decibel hearing loss.

Mini-Canal Hearing Aid   A hearing aid that is between a CIC and canal aid in size.

Moderate Hearing Loss   A forty- to sixty-decibel hearing loss.

Monaural   One Ear.

Most Comfortable Loudness Level (MCL)   The volume or loudness setting that is the most comfortable for a hearing aid user.

Myringotomy   A minor medical procedure in which a small incision is made in the eardrum to drain fluid or infection.

Normal Hearing   Hearing thresholds that are better (less) than twenty decibels.

Occlusion Effect   A change in the acoustical properties of the ear that results from the physical presence of a hearing aid in the ear canal.

This effect can cause a person to feel like he or she is talking inside a barrel. Current hearing aids can sometimes be designed to minimize this effect.

Omni-Directional Microphone   This is the traditional microphone that is built into hearing aids. It picks up sound from all directions.

Open-Platform Hearing Aid   The ultimate in master hearing aids. It can be set for different hearing losses and also has the potential to be reprogrammed to code or filter speech in ways that may not even have been invented yet.

Organ of Corti   The structure that supports the nerve cells in the cochlea.

Ossicles   The malleus, incus, and stapes bones.

Oval Window   The opening between the middle and inner ear where the stapes bone sits.

Pinna   The portion of the ear extending outward beyond the skull. Also called the auricle.

Profound Hearing Loss   A hearing loss greater than one hundred decibels.

Programmable Hearing Aid   Although digital hearing aids are sometimes referred to as being programmable, the term *programmable hearing aid* is generally used to denote a hybrid that has parts of both an analog and a digital hearing aid. It has digital components that allow it to be programmed, but the underlying amplifier is analog.

Receiver   This is the name for the little speaker inside a hearing aid.

Recruitment   A phenomenon where loud sounds may seem every bit as loud for a person with hearing loss as for a person with normal hearing. Recruitment frequently occurs with sensorineural hearing loss.

Residual Inhibition   An effect that sometimes occurs in which tinnitus is reduced or suppressed for a period of time following hearing aid use.

Selective Amplification   The general philosophy of hearing aid fitting that states that the greater the hearing loss at any particular pitch, the more amplification will be needed at that pitch.

Sensorineural Hearing Loss   The type of hearing loss that results when there is damage to the nerve cells in the inner ear.

Severe Hearing Loss   An eighty- to one-hundred-decibel hearing loss.

Stapes   The innermost of the three middle ear bones. Also called the stirrup.

Super Hearing   A fiction that is believed to be fact by a number of people who have hearing loss.

Telecoil   A small device built into many hearing aids that make it easier to hear on the phone. It also serves as an interface between a hearing aid and many assistive listening devices.

Telephone Device for the Deaf (TDD)   This is a special typewriter that plugs into the phone line. Rather than speaking into the phone and listening, a person types and reads. This is also known as a telephone typewriter or text telephone.

Tinnitus   A perceived ringing, roaring, or cricket-like sound in the ear that is not actually present in the outside world.

Tubing   This refers to a small clear tube that carries sound from the body of a behind-the-ear hearing aid to the earmold.

Tympanic Membrane   The eardrum.

Uncomfortable Loudness Level (UCL)   The level at which sounds become uncomfortably loud.

Vent   A small hole that goes through a hearing aid or hearing aid earmold to allow air into the ear. The size of the vent can be modified to change the acoustical properties of a hearing aid.

Vestibular System   The balance portion of the ear. It includes the semicircular canals and vestibule.

Word Discrimination   The ability to distinguish one word from another. The clarity of hearing.

References

Brooks, D. N., R. S. Hallam, P. A. Mellor. 2001. "The Effects on Significant Others of Providing a Hearing Aid to the Hearing-Impaired Partner." *British Journal of Audiology* 35, 3 (June): 165-171.

Cacciatore, F., C. Napoli, P. Abete, E. Marciano, M. Triassi, and F. Rengo. 1999. "Quality of Life Determinants and Hearing Function in an Elderly Population: Osservatorio Geriatrico Campano Study Group." *Gerontology* 45, 6 (November-December): 323-328.

Collins, J. G., and O. T. Thornberry. 1989. "Health Characteristics of Workers by Occupation and Sex: United States, 1983-85." *Advance Data from Vital and Health Statistics* 168:89-1250.

Desai, M., L. A. Pratt, H. Lentzner, and K. N. Robinson. 2001. "Trends in Vision and Hearing among Older Americans." *Aging Trends* 2:1-8.

Kirkwood, D. H. 2002. "Although Opinions Vary, Survey Finds Many Concerned by Consolidation of Dispensing." *Hearing Journal* 55 (3): 21-36.

Kochkin, S. 1990. "MarkeTrak I: Introducing MarkeTrak: The Consumer Tracking Survey of the Hearing Instruments Market." *Hearing Journal* 43 (5): 17-27.

———. 1993. "MarkeTrak III: Higher Hearing Aid Sales Don't Signal Better Market Penetration." *Hearing Journal* 46 (7): 47-54.

———. 1996. "MarkeTrak IV: Ten-Year Trends in the Hearing Aid Market: Has Anything Changed?" *Hearing Journal* 48 (1): 23-34.

Kubler-Ross, E. 1969. *On Death and Dying*. New York: Macmillan Publishing Co.

Mulrow, C. D., C. Aguilar, J. E. Endicott, M. R. Tuley, R. Velez, W. S. Charlip, M. C. Rhodes, J. A. Hill, and L. A. DeNino. 1990. "Quality-of-Life Changes and Hearing Impairment: A Randomized Trial." *Annals of Internal Medicine* 113, 3 (August): 118-194.

Mulrow, C. D., C. Aguilar, J. E. Endicott, R. Velez, M. R. Tuley, W. S. Charlip, and J. A. Hill. 1990. "Associations between Hearing Impairment and the Quality of Life of Elderly Individuals." *Journal of the American Geriatric Society* 38, 1 (January): 45-50.

Mulrow, C. D., M. R. Tuley, and C. Aguilar. 1992. "Sustained Benefits of Hearing Aids." *Journal of Speech and Hearing Research* 35, 6 (December): 1402-1405.

National Council on Aging. 2000. "The Consequences of Untreated Hearing Loss in Older Persons." *Otorhinolaryngology Head and Neck Nursing* 18, 1 (Winter): 12-16.

National Institute on Deafness and Other Communication Disorders. 1989. *A Report of the Task Force on the National Strategic Plan.* Bethesda, Md.: National Institutes of Health.

Ries, P. W. 1994. "Prevalence and Characteristics of Persons with Hearing Trouble: United States, 1990-91." *National Health Survey Series* 10, No. 188.

Russell, J. N., G. E. Hendershot, F. LeClere, L. J. Howie, and M. Adler. 1997. "Trends and Differential Use of Assistive Technology Devices: United States, 1994." *Advance Data from Vital and Health Statistics* 292:1-9.

Weinstein, B. E. 1996. "Treatment Efficacy: Hearing Aids in the Management of Hearing Loss in Adults." *Journal of Speech and Hearing Research* 39:S37-45.

Index

About the Author

John M. Burkey, M.A., is the director of audiology at the Lippy Group for Ear, Nose, and Throat in Warren, Ohio. He is certified by the American Speech-Language-Hearing Association and is a Fellow of the American Academy of Audiology. He has authored, coauthored, and contributed to articles for hearing, hearing aid, and medical journals.